In my work as a holis........ .... naturopath in an energy medicine practice, I am privileged to witness transformation in the lives and health of my clients. But one particular client wasn't experiencing the changes she had hoped for. While she felt wonderful during our sessions, she quickly fell back into old negative patterns after she left and forgot about the changes I suggested. Although she remembered to take her prescription medication every day, she was not using energy medicine on a daily basis.

As I pondered what might help her integrate energy healing into her life, I had a sudden insight during her session:

"Try taking an empty prescription bottle and put a label on it saying 'The Other Medicine: Take Daily' and place it next to your prescription medication. That way when you take your medication in the morning, it will remind you to take your 'other medicine'— energy medicine."

And then it dawned on me..... *The Other Medicine* was the working title of the book I had just finished writing! In the next instant, a vision of the book cover exploded in my mind... the very book cover you are now reading.

I hope this image will help you see that energy-based interventions and practices are indeed medicine, powerful medicine that heals body, mind, and spirit... from the *core* of your being.

THE
OTHER MEDICINE
THAT REALLY WORKS!

How ENERGY MEDICINE Can Help You
Heal in BODY, MIND and SPIRIT

HEIDI DuPREE, RN, CTN

Editorial development and creative design support by Ascent: www.itsyourlifebethere.com

Illustrations by: Kelsey Beerman

Design: Lookout Design, Inc.

Table of Contents

"Holistic Nurses are by far the most competent professionals to help us develop a true Health Care System! It is time for them to rescue us from [the] Medical System..."

—NORMAN SHEALY, M.D., PH.D.

PROLOGUE:

WHAT YOU NEED TO KNOW BEFORE
YOUR HEALING JOURNEY BEGINS

"All truth passes through three stages.
First, it is ridiculed.
Second, it is violently opposed.
Third, it is accepted as being self-evident."

— ARTHUR SCHOPENHAUER

ALL EYES IN THE AUDIENCE were on me as I rose to speak to a local networking group. As the newest member, I had been invited to talk about my book. I came prepared with my "elevator pitch" memorized, that brief summary for getting the point of a book across quickly, meant to be conveyed in the time it takes to ride an elevator. I took a breath and launched into my speech: *"I have written a nonfiction mind-body health book that restores lost knowledge of energy medicine to Western culture by weaving together information from ancient cultures, scientific research, personal stories and case histories of healing from my perspective as both a Western Medicine professional and an Energy Medicine professional. It contains everything you need to know to understand the causes of physical, emotional, mental, and spiritual health issues and the key to healing them in a way that goes beyond symptom elimination into growth and transformation."*

A number of the networkers responded warmly to my brief speech—smiling and nodding. One even shared a positive personal experience from using energy medicine. But a stony-faced woman who identified herself as a scientist avoided eye contact as she spoke: "There's mechanical energy, chemical energy, and thermal energy," she began. "But there's no such thing as an energy field. And the idea of a connection between energy and health is nonsense. People who believe such things are idiots. *Idiots!"*

After her tirade, everyone's attention in the room turned back to me, looking for my reaction. But my reaction to this public and personal attack was not readily visible. It was happening on a subtle, energetic level, even though the effects were not subtle at all to me! The normally smooth hum of my energy systems became instantly harsh and chaotic, creating jagged waveforms that initiated a cascade of physiological responses—a tightening in my stomach, blood rushing to my face, and an internal shaking imperceptible to the outside observer.

Although this was not my first such public experience, I was still stunned into silence. Having my work attacked by a scientist should not have come as a surprise, however, given the current state of scientific publishing. According to astronomer Halton Arp, "The tradition of 'peer review' articles published in professional journals has degenerated into almost total censorship. The result is real investigative science is mostly now an underground activity."

Indeed, much of the study of science has historically been about verifying already known concepts, not exploring new territory. In her rebuke of energy medicine, the scientist at the networking meeting was referring to physical, measurable, or *veritable* energy, while dismissing subtle, immeasurable, or *putative* energy. It has only been the pioneering scientists willing to brave harassment who have begun to do the research that documents subtle energy and the energetic structures of the body, research that this particular scientist was undoubtedly unaware of. I was also once unaware of this, even though modern documentation of ancient wisdom regarding energy medicine began over a century ago.

It wasn't until after the meeting, when I had time to process the event and recover my energy that I recalled how I was once like the scientist, dismissive of energy concepts....

While studying to become a registered nurse in the late 1970s, one of my instructors invited a guest speaker to give a presentation and demonstration on "therapeutic touch." The nurse speaker claimed that without actually touching a person, but rather by making contact with the "energy field" around the body with her hands, she could speed wound healing and relieve pain.

The presentation lasted an hour, but I think I stopped listening after about five minutes. If there was such a thing as an energy field around the human body, then why couldn't I see it? Why hadn't I heard of it before? If only one hour out of my four-year education—just weeks prior to graduation—was devoted to the existence of this field, then it must not be very important. Years later I would take this presentation as a sign that the conventional medical field was, even then, beginning to accept the validity of energy-based healing therapies, but at the time, all I could think was—*why is this information being tossed in at the last minute?* Why was the instructor wasting our time?

The available programs in nursing at that time were based on the Western medical model of healthcare. It was all I knew.

The idea that one could facilitate healing in another with nothing but their hands seemed ludicrous. I couldn't imagine how such a presentation had any place in a respectable university nursing curriculum. I glanced around the room at the other nursing students, studying their faces, trying to gage their reaction. Did they also find this presentation strange and irrelevant?

Everything in my education and limited experience as a twenty-one-year-old told me that healing was accomplished through Western medical treatment—surgery and prescription drugs aimed at eradicating symptoms of disease. While I was taught in nursing school to consider the whole person and take every aspect of their lives into account in their care, the *basis* of that care was a focus on illness and disease. My job as a nurse was to care for sick people and teach them how to *manage* their disease, *eat* for their disease, and *take medications* for their disease.

When the presentation ended I felt irritated. This silliness about energy and waving hands over the body had taken away precious time needed for practicing important skills—like giving intramuscular injections, calculating drug dosages, or changing dressings.

But even as I studied the Western model, something else was already beginning to trouble me.

Yes, this brief exposure to an alternative therapy—so-called "energy work"—left me with a negative impression. But truthfully, I also felt something vaguely unsettling about my nursing education. Even as I was rejecting non-conventional therapies, I also had the sense that maybe Western medicine *wasn't* the only approach, or even the best approach. But at the time, I was too immersed in Western medical culture to pay attention to these feelings.

More than ten years would pass before that unsettled feeling about the limitations of Western medicine emerged again. As my life began to fall apart in my early 30s, I had to face the reality that the model I had staked my career on couldn't help me. With the realization that my previously accepted view of reality was only an illusion, I thought I was losing my mind. *"You're going to think I'm weird,"* I said to the psychotherapist I consulted for help.

As I began to heal, I connected with my life's purpose—energy healing and the emerging field of energy medicine. But even though I knew what I was meant to do with my life, at first I would stammer and say, "Well, *you're going to think I'm weird,* but I practice energy healing therapies," when someone asked me what I did for a living.

I no longer devalue who I am or what I do with those words. I no longer use those words because I know energy healing is grounded in traditions that date back as far as there are records. I no longer use those words because I know about the scientific discoveries of the last hundred years that validate energy healing therapies. And I no longer use those words because I have healed enough to know better.

Even though I no longer use those words, I can still be triggered by certain situations—such as a stranger referring to me as an idiot in public. In the past, such an attack would have knocked me flat, precipitating illness and a retreat to my bed. The fact that I could see this experience for what it was—an opportunity for growth—and use it as a vehicle for continuing the transformation of old negative beliefs about worthiness and safety is a testament to my own healing journey.

However, the clients coming to me aren't there yet, and

perhaps you aren't either. Many of the individuals I work with have just awakened to a strange world where everything seems upside down. They come to me vulnerable, apprehensive, and lost. These newly awakened souls say to me, *"You're going to think I'm weird."*

And I say, *"I most definitely do not think you are weird."* Far from it. I see *you*, a being ready to let go of its garbage, ready to evolve, but not knowing how. I see a butterfly emerging from its cocoon, beginning to open its wings... and what I see is *beautiful*.

And I think how amazing it is that I have been entrusted with this opportunity to witness the unfolding of another human being, and to share what I've learned with you in this book.

So dear reader, it's OK with me if you think I'm weird, but I won't think that of you. Come along with me and let's explore the nature of life and other "lost" knowledge of health and healing.

— 1 —

ENERGETIC BEGINNINGS

STORIES OF HEALING & WHAT'S IN IT FOR YOU

Joy and woe are woven fine,
A clothing for the soul divine.
Under every grief and pines
Runs a joy with silken twine.

—WILLIAM BLAKE

JOCELYN WAS A WOMAN desperate for help. I took in her disheveled appearance; her uncombed hair, lack of makeup, wrinkled clothes. Her pale, blotchy skin and the dark circles under her eyes spoke of her extreme stress, which she confirmed with the statement, "I'm at the end of my rope." Even though she was anxious, depressed and unable to sleep, Jocelyn had stopped taking her prescription medications for anxiety, depression and insomnia because they made her feel "half dead."

There was more. Jocelyn hated her job and had no idea what her purpose in life was. Her home was at risk of foreclosure due to financial difficulties. And she had just broken up with her boyfriend—another failed relationship in a series of confusing connections with men who were either abusive or not available.

"This is not how I expected my life to turn out. Life has been such a huge disappointment," she said through tears.

When Western medical treatment failed to help, Jocelyn decided to come to me. She admitted that she doubted I could help her either. But in my experience I knew a part of her had hope, or she wouldn't have made the appointment. "I probably sound pathetic to you," she concluded, dabbing at her eyes with a tissue.

After I finished asking Jocelyn questions about her health history, and listening to her concerns, I invited her to lie on her back on a padded table in my healing treatment room, the same kind of table used for massages. Sessions take place in a small womb-like room with high windows and a soothing mural painted on one wall. Cool, dappled light filtering through shrubs just outside the windows gives the room a relaxed feel. As Jocelyn slipped off her shoes I lit an aromatherapy candle scented with spices from Madagascar and turned a white noise machine on low to occupy my left brain, freeing up my intuitive right brain.

I made Jocelyn comfortable with a pillow under her knees and covered her with a quilt because people often become chilled when they reach a deep state of relaxation.

Here in this small room, the truth is Jocelyn was not just lying back on a table but stepping across the borders of a new frontier in healthcare.

Honoring the Person

"I'm going to start by supporting your feet in my hands and tune in to your system," I said to Jocelyn. "Would that be all right?" I asked.

This is how I begin all my sessions, by gently laying my hands on the most non-threatening body part, the feet. While I'm at someone's feet, I ground and center myself by focusing on my breathing and my connection to the earth through the sensation of my feet pressing down on the floor. In this position, I begin to connect with the client on a deep level. In this state, I silently say a prayer for healing.

As I moved to slide my hands under Jocelyn's ankles, I noticed right away that her body was so tense and rigid that her heels were not even touching the table. I looked at the quilt covering her body and could see that, over her chest and abdomen it was barely rising and falling. Her breathing was so shallow I could barely detect movement.

To begin the healing process, I guided Jocelyn in being present in the moment by taking some slow, deep breaths. "Imagine that you can *breathe* in the energy from my hands. With each breathe you take in, you are breathing in *energy*. And with each exhalation, you are breathing out anxiety and stress. With each breath, you are settling more and more into your body, sinking into the table, going deeper, and deeper," I said softly.

When I drew Jocelyn's attention to the tension in her body, she was surprised. She hadn't noticed these things about herself. Often the people who seek my help are out of touch with the state of their physical body—such as shallow breathing, shoulders pulled up to their ears, or clenched jaw—even as they vividly describe certain other symptoms or problems—such as stomach aches, headaches or depression. But as they lay on the healing table, and I begin to direct their attention to their body, they notice such sensations as the pressure in their head, constriction in their throat, heaviness in their chest, tightness in their belly.

As Jocelyn began to relax, I explained the interactive nature of my work and that she could talk to me and ask questions. She didn't have to lie still and be perfectly quiet! Then I moved my hand to her belly to keep her awareness in her body as I explored her emotional state and self-concepts.

"It is helpful for me as I work with you to know what you believe about yourself. Some people find it very difficult to say, *I completely love and accept myself.* Would that be easy for you to say, or difficult?" I asked.

As is frequently the case with many of my clients, Jocelyn had great difficulty saying those words. Although she was caring toward others, her judgment of herself was harsh. She expressed love and patience for her children, but reserved none for herself.

"Why can't I just pull myself together?" she asked. And she wanted to know how many sessions it would take for me to "fix" her.

I knew that if Jocelyn wanted to heal her life, she would have to go much deeper than symptoms. And she would need to understand that I had no more power to "fix" her than did the physicians she had given up on.

Because the power to heal and transform herself from the inside-out was already within her.

This is something I discovered many years before—a basic but radical truth about healing.

The Dark Night of the Soul

Before I finish Jocelyn's story, I want to tell you how I came to do the work I am doing. And I want you to know that I would never view any of the clients who come to see me when conventional medicine fails to help as "pathetic," because if they are, then in comparison I was once a basket case! I do this work from an experiential place, as I was once the one lying on the table. In my work, I bring my experiences—having gone on this same healing journey myself—as well as the skills developed as a professional nurse, my training as an energy medicine therapist, or "healer," and my education in traditional naturopathy.

I use the term *energy medicine* rather than the traditional word *healer* because energy medicine more accurately reflects this emerging, scientifically-validated field. I also make this distinction because the term healer implies that I can "heal" people. As we shall see, a healing therapist or practitioner *facilitates* healing.

Sometimes the clients in my professional healing practice find it difficult to imagine that I was once in their shoes, and with good reason, because I'm not the same person that I was. I once completely lacked self-awareness and self-compassion. I would bend over backwards for others, but I didn't think I deserved the same. I continually gave to others from a place of emptiness. The roots of this self-rejection and emptiness began early in life.

Throughout my childhood, my father's job transfers necessitated a number of interstate moves. I lived on both the East and West coasts, as well as in the mid-West, and each relocation brought with it culture shock as I tried to adjust to different customs and expectations.

Shy and reserved by nature, the moves compounded my sense of isolation, repeatedly taking me away from the few friends I had. We usually lived far from extended family and any supportive family friendships we formed were repeatedly severed each time we relocated.

The moves were especially difficult for me because my attachment to my parents was insecure. By this I mean I didn't feel unconditionally loved or accepted for who I was. And I felt unable to have a voice, to express my own anger, or to be my authentic self.

I proceeded through life unaware of the full impact of these early difficulties, acquiring the typical milestones in an almost robotic state. By my early thirties, my life had all the outward signs of success; a happy ten-year marriage to my husband, Robert, our two wonderful children Jonathan and Monica, a new home, and a job I enjoyed as a clinical nurse working in obstetrics and lactation consulting.

The stability in my life at this time served as the unconscious signal that I was ready to enter the *dark night of the soul*— although I did not know it at the time. References to this life phase appear in spiritual traditions throughout the world. It is a time of intense growth that can be marked by suffering and a sense of hopelessness, where your worst nightmare seems to be coming true. This is followed by transformation and higher levels of consciousness.

At first, slight cracks began to form in my perfectly constructed facade. On the surface I was the happy wife and mother living in a pretty white house with a manicured front lawn. But anxiety and depression were making it more and more difficult to keep up the appearance of normalcy. I existed in a low-energy state filled with shame, guilt, and fear. As discontent began seeping more and more into my everyday life, I became increasingly depressed and spiraled into self-loathing. If life was so grand, why did I feel so empty and dead inside?

I longed for more out of life, more out of my relationships, and more meaning in my work. However, to express any dissatisfaction with a life I had worked so hard to create was unthinkable.

So I tried to keep it suppressed. But the anxiety could not be suppressed with overeating or numbed through hyperactivity.

I manufactured chaos in my life to feel alive—impossible deadlines and frenetic activity. Throwing myself into wallpapering every wall of our new house, I worked late into the night in a manic state, even wallpapering the inside of closets. Years later, the process of removing all that wallpaper would become a healing ritual, a way to process and release the trauma from this very difficult time in my life. But at the time, the frantic pace was all I had to keep from feeling the huge empty hole inside of me. And it only grew worse, evolving into panic attacks. Bewildered, Robert bore witness to my disintegration. Like a deer caught in headlights, frozen in panic and terror, I would hyperventilate until I nearly passed out.

Along with the panic attacks, memories of childhood sexual trauma began to surface as confusing fragments. I remembered in detail an apartment I had never lived in, and physical characteristics of a man I had no conscious memory of. It wasn't until a transpersonal psychotherapist guided me into a meditative state that I was able to access the full memory of being molested by a babysitter's boyfriend when I was between two and three years old.

Although I had been unaware of this sexual trauma, the signs had been there all along. As a teenager, I had felt as prickly and unapproachable as a porcupine, recoiling from touch; issues that followed me into adulthood, along with severe depressive episodes, an eating disorder, low self-esteem, sexual dysfunction, infertility, and poor body awareness.

When I think back to these earlier times in my life, I can barely recognize who I was. It was as if I was sleepwalking through life, going through the motions of living without being fully present.

I existed in my head with little awareness of my body. My mind was an endless loop of negative thoughts disconnected from a sea of negative emotions. A massage therapist commented that it was as if my body was made of stone. I didn't understand what she was talking about, because I felt nothing. I went through each day unaware of the layers of deep tension I carried. I was only aware of how tired I was; an all-consuming tiredness that would eventually be diagnosed as chronic fatigue syndrome.

Worst of all was the feeling of being alone and cut off. While I held a mental belief in God, I had no real sense of spirituality and religion had no meaning to me. I felt lost, trapped, and angry at myself, angry at the body that had betrayed me, angry at the physicians who couldn't help me, angry at God for abandoning me, and jealous of others who appeared to have a normal life. Like Jocelyn, I had no idea where to go for answers and was unaware that my feelings of disconnection, emptiness and exhaustion were due to major disruptions in my energy systems.

This unawareness had its consequences. In this unaddressed state I developed cancer, gallstones, and autoimmune disease. And those health consequences created even more energetic disruption.

The process of building our family through many years of infertility treatment had also taken a huge toll, and it was not over. While infertility may not seem like that big a challenge, it is widely regarded as a major life crisis of similar magnitude to a diagnosis of cancer or HIV infection, regardless of whether the family already has children. Having had both cancer and infertility, I can attest to the parallels between them. Both impact every aspect of your life, and if treated with Western medicine, can involve lengthy, invasive treatment with less than promising success rates.

Although the cancer scare seemed behind me, I carried on the infertility struggle like a weary soldier, engaged in a seemingly endless battle, a war that left me bitter. Why had this happened to us? What was the point of all the suffering?

From Skeptic to Expert

I think most people today are aware of the existence of alternatives to conventional or "allopathic" medicine, but at the time I began having panic attacks, I had no such awareness. It wasn't until the transpersonal psychotherapist I began seeing suggested I consult with a healing practitioner that I even remembered the nursing school presentation on therapeutic touch, when the seeds of doubt about my career path into Western medicine were first planted. My sense of trust in my therapist coupled with growing disillusionment with allopathic medicine both as a clinical nurse and an infertility patient led me to reconsider my earlier dismissive stance. I could no longer ignore the unsettled feeling that was growing and cracking apart my life as I knew it.

I began to realize that my identity had been built on illusions and false beliefs about myself as a victim, and a person unworthy of love and acceptance—separate from God, from others, and from the flow of life. Like a house built of cards, those illusions were crashing down. Everything that I thought I was, everything that I knew about myself was false. I didn't even know who I was anymore.

As I worked with healing professionals, I began to grasp that healing wasn't about resisting, suppressing, or eliminating distressing symptoms. I would come to understand that I wasn't going to find my answers by staying busy and distracted, or in consulting allopathic professionals—because my answers were *within*. The very thing I had been fighting against with all my might was a message from deep within myself—the doorway to a happier, healthier, and more meaningful life. And with that insight, I began to emerge from the dark night.

Coming into the Light

When I began my path into healing, the most I hoped for would be to "overcome" infertility and other health issues. While my health issues and infertility did resolve, the journey would be so much more; taking me to deeper places within that I didn't know existed and becoming the opportunity to heal my whole being. When I fully accepted myself, and the layers of garbage that I carried began to clear, my inner light was revealed.

Through the traumas of my life I was given an almost unimaginable gift—the opportunity to heal *to the core*. And from that core, the changes rippled out through every aspect of my life. Coming into the light transformed my health, career, relationships, and belief systems; including a new understanding of healing beyond the biomechanical level I was taught.

Jocelyn's transition into the light began with an awareness of the impact of her own traumatic experiences from her past. During her childhood, her sister's sudden, unexpected death preceded the disintegration of her family. Her loving parents, incapacitated by grief, all but abandoned her and her brother. With the light gone in their family, she became the target for her brother's anger. He terrorized her, sometimes locking her in a closet. While she had been in psychotherapy for years, she hadn't been fully aware of the deep impact of these traumatic childhood events on every part of her being.

Although Jocelyn was skeptical of my suggestion that these past events were at the root of her current emotional difficulties, she admitted she had suffered from claustrophobia for years and could barely tolerate my hands laid on her body because it made her feel trapped.

"So you think that has something to do with what happened in my childhood?" she asked.

"Absolutely," I replied.

"But we were just being kids. My parents were doing the best they could under the circumstances."

"I'm sure they were, but that doesn't take away from the fact that you were deeply affected and are still dealing with those effects."

I could see what she had difficulty seeing, that her current state of being was a reflection of past traumatic experiences. I've worked with people who range from suicidal to the new mother who feels depleted; from the completely disabled, to the person who has developed a rash. In every case, whether they were aware of it or not, there was more going on than what the client initially presented to me. Under the surface were unresolved events or issues from the past.

All of us carry disruptions from past events of our lives. Until these disruptions are dealt with, our past traumas will continue to create physical, emotional, mental, and spiritual difficulties in the present. While there is no need to *relive* the past, we may need to *revisit* the past.

As our work together began releasing the effects of the traumas on every level, I saw the light come back in Jocelyn's eyes. The deep tension that she had held throughout her body slowly dissipated and she was able to sleep again. She began to wear brighter colors, got a new hairstyle, and her skin glowed. She found her purpose in life in the teaching profession and the last I heard from her she was taking evening classes for a provisional teaching license.

A few months later an email arrived from Jocelyn full of excitement over all the recent positive changes in her life. She thought she would never have a home again after losing her house to foreclosure, but now she had a beautiful new house to live in for a low monthly rent, provided by a family member who bought it as an investment. The teaching job of her dreams that she hadn't even applied for was offered to her. And she was most excited about a new relationship with a man who was as interested in her as she was in him. He was kind, caring and supportive of her life, qualities she had never experienced before in a relationship.

In learning to love herself, Jocelyn had attracted love in her life. As she changed on the inside, those changes were reflected in her outer life. The long road she had taken since first awakening, leaving her job, breaking up with her boyfriend, and losing her house—all while facing her fears and struggling to trust in her healing process—had brought her to an amazing new life. And it had all happened in surprising and unexpected ways.

"It's as if I've come into the light, after a lifetime of residing in the darkness," read Jocelyn's email.

Now I don't want to imply that Jocelyn was "done." Like life itself, healing is a process that is never really "finished," and as some would argue, does not even end with death. As we shall learn, healing is a growth process, not a destination.

What about You?

Are you feeling lost, confused, overwhelmed, disconnected, or exhausted—like your life is falling apart? Perhaps you've read self-help books that encourage "conquering" or "surviving" your issues, but you are interested in more than just surviving and have a sense that healing is not about fighting and resisting. You may have had negative experiences with Western medical treatment, or are beginning to realize that our current conventional medical system doesn't have all the answers.

If you have heard of energy healing therapies, they may have sounded so foreign that it caused some apprehension. Or you might think that energy-based modalities are only an occasional indulgence for temporary relaxation and stress relief. While the process of healing does include stress reduction and enhanced relaxation, a more accurate description of energy medicine interventions and practices is deep physical, emotional, mental, and spiritual healing that occurs at the core of our being.

When I began studying books about energy healing, I didn't understand any of it. It was as if the books were written in a foreign language. These works contained a lot of information about specific energy healing techniques written by authors who had always been aware of energy systems and their intuitive abilities. But as an individual with no prior knowledge of energy healing, no understanding of energy systems, and little awareness of intuition, these books had left me confused and wondering— *how exactly does energy medicine work?*

As you read about Jocelyn's healing and mine, perhaps you're also wondering how energy medicine works, and how such transformational healing took place in our lives. To answer those questions, I invite you to go on a journey with me, a journey of healing through empowering information. I will illustrate this information through stories of many interesting people from all walks of life, some of whom may remind you of yourself. And I will weave summaries of scientific discoveries that validate energy medicine throughout this book. This is information I wish had been available to me at the beginning of my journey, presented in a way that is accessible to anyone—from the initiate to the advanced student of energy medicine.

I have written this book for you and for the people I see each day who are in physical and emotional pain, who are plagued with repetitive negative thoughts, or who are experiencing a spiritual crisis. They are being told there is nothing wrong with them and that there is nothing that can be done for them. Or they are being given medications that don't help or actually make them worse. Many have felt hopeless and don't know where to turn.

Each day I am honored to be a part of miracles large and small happening in the lives of my clients. I have seen what has been deemed impossible become possible. But in my practice, I can only help a few people a day. Through the medium of this book, I hope to help many more.

In the pages of this book, I will act as your healing guide. With over thirty years of experience working in healthcare, half in Western medicine and half in energy medicine, I am fluent in the language of both and can serve as your interpreter. But beyond that, my ability to be your guide comes through having experienced the journey of healing myself, and doing the "inner work" required to facilitate healing in others.

It is no accident that you have picked this book. If you have opened these pages, something in your life is calling to you. As your guide, I will show you how the problem that you are trying to get rid of may, in itself, be the pathway to whole person healing—the path to happiness, harmony, peace, vibrancy, freedom, and wholeness. If it feels like cracks are forming in your life, those cracks may be what is needed for the light within to reveal itself.

And I consider it an honor to join you on your path of life for a short while.

*   *   *

When we reach the end of our time together, you will have the information you need to live a physically, emotionally, mentally, and spiritually healing way of life, and a more complete understanding of the healing process.

Along with a list of recommended reading resources to help you continue your journey at the end of this book, you will also find a "capsule" of energy medicine at the end of each chapter—in the form of word-energy affirmations to support your journey. This is the same way that I end many of my client sessions, with an affirmation to continue the integration process after the session is over. Though I'm unable to offer you an affirmation personalized just for you, I have used my intuition to guide me in what would be helpful. You can also use your fingers to tap on the acupoints depicted in the illustration in the appendix while you say these affirmations to yourself.

It is my sincere hope that this book will inspire you
to find your own path to personal healing.

PART ONE:

SCIENCE & ANATOMY ESSENTIALS

Understanding Energy as the Basis of Life

"A human being is a part of a whole, called by us 'universe',
a part limited in time and space. He experiences himself, his
thoughts and feelings as something separated from the rest...
a kind of optical delusion of his consciousness.
Our task must be to free ourselves from this prison
by widening our circle of compassion to embrace all
living creatures and the whole of nature in its beauty."

—ALBERT EINSTEIN

~2~

ENERGY SCIENCE

*"As the new physics unfolds, we are finding that its
new laws support some of the universal tenets of religion:
the reality and survival of the soul, the power of prayer,
and the existence of other dimensions."*

—CLAUDE SWANSON, PH.D.

"I FEEL STUCK IN MY LIFE," said Katie. "I just can't seem to move forward with anything. I'm not sure I've ever recovered from cancer treatment three years ago. Do you think you can help me?"

Katie, a pleasant woman in her 40s with thick brown hair that swept across the top of her round face, came for an appointment after noticing positive changes in a friend who was also my client. As I observed her, I was struck by a deep sense of emptiness beneath her congenial surface.

From the moment I sat down with Katie to talk about her issues, I was in a relaxed, calm state, fully present in the moment. By being completely focused on Katie and listening with all my senses, thinking only of her and what her body-mind was telling me, I was in a meditative-type state. I was now prepared for what was to come next.

A Conduit

I remained in this state of deep listening with an open heart as Katie reclined on my healing table and I gently laid my hands on her, continuing to open my intuition. Then came the part that is often harder for people to understand or accept, given the lack of knowledge about the energetic nature of life that permeates every aspect of our society, including healthcare. As my hands lay on Katie, *healing energy* began to flow through my hands. Now I don't mean that I was giving away *my* energy. In my first practice session as a healing student, I actually did that, and felt terrible afterwards—completely drained. What I do mean is that I allowed energy to flow *through* me, rather than *from* me.

As a healing therapist, I do not believe I am the source of healing energy. Rather, I am the conduit; the channel through which the energy flows to the client. In *Outrageous Openness: Letting the Divine Take the Lead,* astrologer Tosha Silver writes "Life changes radically if you know you're a conduit for what wishes to happen as opposed to the one making it all occur."

Through her study of individuals ill from HIV infection, Stanford Medical School psychiatrist Dr. Elizabeth Targ confirmed that this approach to healing is the most effective. Sick individuals in her study who were exposed to healing practitioners who thought of themselves as a channel, rather than the source of the healing, experienced the greatest improvement in their condition.

Softening my hands so they molded to Katie's body, I begin to relax and listen. By becoming the neutral receiver of her energy, impressions began to form—mental images, descriptive words in my mind, and physical sensations in my hands such as tingling, denseness, or diffuseness. Staying open and relaxed allowed my own energy "field" to be free of any resistance, which in turn allowed the client's energy to freely express and reveal its patterns.

In *Craniosacral Therapy and the Energetic Body*, energy medicine and craniosacral therapy teacher Roger Gilchrist refers to this as "negotiating space," a way of being that requires a healing practitioner have a good relationship with their own self, and to accept the client exactly as they are. Gilchrist writes, "This willingness to meet another human being entirely on her own terms immediately invokes the quality of genuineness, because we have to be fully who we are in order to do so." In this energetic environment, the healing process can begin to unfold.

SESSION NOTES:

Connecting with a client in this manner creates a "closed circuit," a term usually associated with electrical systems, meaning an uninterrupted path for the flow of electrical current. In living systems, a closed circuit can be created by connecting energy with another person or living being, achieved through touching the body or energy field of another with both hands. Closed systems of energy are also created when a group of people join hands, or if you place your hands on your own body for self-healing.

Under the laws of physics, in a group of two or more the energy of a closed system tends to even itself out. In other words, the energies of individuals in a system will become synchronized to the most stable energy. Similarly, it has been documented that both the heart and brain rhythms of two persons sitting quietly and facing each other with eyes closed will synchronize, an effect that is enhanced if they become physically connected by holding a wire between them. This natural process of "syncing up" is called *entrainment.*

As I connected with Katie's energy field, I noticed that her energy rhythms were barely perceptible to my senses, almost suppressed. Over the course of the session, our energies would begin to synchronize to the most stable state, which given my training as a healing practitioner, is mine. But at first, her energy field felt dense to my hands.

"I'm getting images in my mind's eye of your energy field. It looks and feels like a large, dense, dark block the size of a refrigerator," I said.

Katie laughed at my refrigerator analogy, saying "My body does feel like a big solid block. I've had problems with weight my whole life, but it's more than that. It's this stuck feeling."

As I continued to share energy through my hands, Katie became aware of tension in her lower abdomen that she described as being shaped like a ball the size of a grapefruit.

"Bring your focus to this ball-like tension in your abdomen," I instructed her. "Breathe as if you are sending your breath right into the tension while observing it. Does it have a color? What else do you notice about it?"

"It feels hollow, and dark."

"Let yourself slip into it, as if it were a pool of water."

"I'm trying to make it go away."

"For the purposes of this exercise, it's best not to do that. Let it fully express itself, even if it needs to get bigger or tighter. Let go of any resistance. Just surrender to it."

"I feel like I'm on the CAT scan table. I can taste the chemo-therapy drugs."

"Good, what else do you notice?"

"The ball of tension is getting smaller, but I feel fear that I could get sick again. My chest and throat are getting tight."

"You're doing great. Stay with it. Keep breathing and sending your breathe into the tension."

The Energetic Difference

By the end of the session, Katie's fear released and her tension dissolved. She noticed a feeling of lightness throughout her body, a foreign sensation that surprised her. To my awareness, her field felt less dense and appeared brighter, and her energy rhythms were more alive—smoother and more harmonious. I stopped the flow of energy between us by breaking the closed circuit for healing simply by removing my hands and ending the intention for healing.

After the session, Katie made another appointment, but admitted she felt confused on how exactly energy healing had worked. As she walked out the door, she asked "Do you think you can explain to me next time how this works? I don't understand what made my body feel lighter."

I could understand her confusion. To answer that question properly would have taken hours. But it got me thinking. It isn't easy being an intuitive energy medicine therapist in a culture where logic and linear thinking rules. My intuition guides me in how to work with my client's issues, but explaining it is another matter.

When Katie left that day I thought of a skeptical client I once worked with who at the end of his first and only session said, "That was very relaxing, but I'm not so sure about this 'energy' thing." Or Helen, who said, "My appointments with you are really helping, but I think it's important for me to also have treatment that is scientific." And then there was Brooke, who said, "I stopped coming to you for a while because my family and friends were so against it. They think you're a witch."

Our families want us to be safe, but sometimes their fearful efforts to protect can block us from getting the help we need. I can understand why people are apprehensive. I remember back in the 70s when individuals who jogged and shunned processed, artificial food in favor of whole and organic, and those who used consciousness-raising practices such as transcendental meditation, were portrayed as "health nuts" that had fallen for a crazy fad. Today the health benefits of exercise, natural foods and the use of meditation are widely known and considered mainstream. We have always fought and resisted new ideas. It takes time for information to become accepted and integrated into our culture.

The more I thought about Katie's question, the concerns of others, and my own difficulty explaining to people "what I do," the importance of addressing these apprehensions and misunderstandings became clear. Energy medicine is not considered mainstream and hasn't been recognized for what it is—*healthcare*—at least not yet. But I have begun to realize that part of my work is to raise the public's awareness by presenting the growing body of research of the last century and summarizing the work of scientists for those who aren't aware of it, for those who know it but can't articulate it, and for those who are part way there but need help to get the rest of the way. Building a bridge of understanding and trust with the clients who come to me for healing requires delving into the advances in scientific research that validate and help explain the basis of energy medicine.

As I worked with Katie, I shared with her some of this research. We discussed important events in history that influenced the direction of science and caused energy-based treatments to nearly go extinct in the U.S. As Katie learned about the scientific basis of energy healing, consciousness, and intuition, she had a greater understanding of the changes that were unfolding in her life. She became an active participant in her healing process, adopting energy-based self-care practices that will be detailed in chapter 14. As she did, the release of layers of disturbances in her energy systems and long-suppressed emotions was accelerated, leading to health and happiness.

I would like to share this information with you as well. To begin, we need to go back in time to see where we strayed from the original intentions for healthcare in the U.S., and how our American system of medical care got so far off track. Like Katie, you may find this information interesting and integral to your own healing. I will only be scratching the surface in terms of the research that is available and growing every day. For additional information, I encourage you to consult the books listed in the recommended reading section of the appendix.

Building a Bridge

Not only is it difficult to explain energy healing because of the emphasis on logic over intuition in our culture, but also because, like a majority of Americans, I grew up after 1910 and before the early 1990's, a time period in our nation's history when many energy-based healing modalities were lost and became virtually unknown. By 1923, therapies that had once flourished in the U.S., such as radioesthesia, and electromagnetic therapies, disappeared and all but two of the twenty-two schools of homeopathy closed.

This period was also marked by an ever-increasing dependence on communicating through written and spoken language, disconnecting us from our inherent intuitive abilities to communicate through sensing energy.

As human beings, we haven't lost our intuition; we just stopped paying attention. And even when we do become aware of our ability to sense energy, all too often we allow others to talk us out of what we already know because we don't trust our instincts or don't have the language to articulate it. I think of it as claiming your own "inner authority" when you make a choice to have faith in your intuition.

Perhaps you have been aware of this disconnect between something you just *know*, having the words to explain it, and being comfortable expressing it? Have you ever prefaced expression of your intuition with "this is going to sound crazy," or "you're going to think I'm weird"? When we label intuitive information as "weird" or "crazy," we are devaluing our intuition.

You may have noticed that just being in the presence of certain people or certain situations makes you feel uncomfortable, unsafe, agitated, drained, or energized—even if the person is a stranger who you know nothing about. Or you may have sensed when someone was watching you or when they entered the same room, even if they were out of your line of sight. You may have kept such observations to yourself, or dismissed them outright. These experiences are not just happening in the mind; our body and energy systems are responding.

Whether we realize it or not, we all have this basic ability to sense and read energy—it's even in our language. When we speak of thoughts, ideas, or beliefs that "resonate" with us, or when we refer to a person or place giving off a "bad vibe"—these are all energetic descriptions.

The lack of knowledge of energy medicine and energy as the basis of life in our culture can be traced back to the publication in the United States in 1910 of the *Flexner Report*. This pivotal study of medical education by professional educator Abraham Flexner of the Carnegie Foundation for Advancement of Teaching recommended improvement in standards for medical training and practice, setting a mandate that they be more "scientific." Max Planck fathered the field of quantum physics in 1900 with the publication of his theories on the nature of reality as probabilities and tendencies, and Albert Einstein published his theory of relativity in 1905, which advanced that time and space are not linear and the observer cannot be separated from what is observed; but these discoveries were not considered in determining the science our healthcare system would be based on.

Stay with me for a brief survey of how we got to where we are today in terms of our Western beliefs about the mind, the body and how we heal.

The Interrupted Lineage of Energy Medicine

Our world view since the 1630s has been shaped by the philosophy of René Descartes, who saw the universe as a "great machine," and by the laws of Sir Isaac Newton, another mathematician and philosopher-physicist whose work provided an explanation for how the world works. The laws formulated by Newton are mechanistic and impersonal in describing a physical world that is separate from self. When Descartes was unable to prove the validity of spiritual concepts using the scientific methodology of his day, science and spirituality were separated into two realms. The influence of these philosophers persists in our society to this day, creating an illusion of separation seen in our belief systems—which ultimately impacts our health.

The theories of Newtonian physics *do* have applications on the macro level, for instance when it comes to the movement of planets. But on the micro level of atomic and subatomic particles, the laws of Newtonian physics simply *lose relevance*.

In the last century, discoveries of the behavior and properties of subatomic particles have turned Newtonian physics on its head.

You were likely taught that our world is made up of solid building blocks of matter. If you put your hand in front of your face, it would appear to be a solid mass of cells that make up your flesh and bone. But if you looked at your hand under an electron microscope, you would see that it is actually made of vibrating energy.

It wasn't until I furthered my education by studying traditional naturopathy after two decades of practicing as a nurse that I even heard of quantum physics and the many other research advances that had made the science of my nursing education obsolete. Why hadn't I heard of these advances, even though I was working in a field with direct applications for the findings of quantum physics?

To answer that question we have to go back to the Flexner Report.

In response to the report's recommendations, medical curriculum and practices were required to conform to protocols based on mainstream science. Despite the publication of Einstein's theory of relativity and the beginning research discoveries of quantum physicists, the prevailing science of the U.S. in 1910 was, and still is to a large degree, based on Newtonian theories. And once medical practices were set on the Newtonian path in the West, they continued in that direction, creating a healthcare system economically dependent on technology and a mechanistic model, where disease is attributed to a malfunction in a linear biochemical process.

In a post-Flexner Report world, healing systems based on the belief that energy fields direct our health and physiology, such as homeopathy, naturopathy, and chiropractic were either marginalized, or all but died out in the U.S., while the emphasis in medical training became biochemical drugs.

Despite a wealth of new discoveries in quantum physics, cellular biology, and electrical engineering, little of this new knowledge has been integrated into Western medical standards of practice. Although allopathy does use quantum technology to read energy fields through the use of CAT scans, MRIs, and PET scans, most Western medical practices, including the use of prescription drugs, are still based on a Newtonian model, where the body is seen as a machine made up of separate parts and information is thought to be transmitted in a linear manner.

While chiropractic has experienced resurgence and expansion since winning a 1990 medical monopoly court case against the American Medical Association, the profession of naturopathy has been split apart.

In the 1950's, in an attempt to move out of the fringes and gain acceptance, a hybrid of allopathy and naturopathy was created called "medical naturopathy," where practitioners perform invasive procedures and diagnose and treat illness, a departure from the non-medical (as defined in the West) and non-invasive philosophical roots of naturopathy. The result has been a healing profession pitted against itself, with separate schools for traditional naturopathy and medical naturopathy, and separate accrediting and certifying bodies that do not necessarily recognize each other.

Medical naturopaths have been using legal means to create a monopoly in the practice of naturopathy and to secure their place as primary care physicians, a role critics claim they are inadequately prepared for. Traditional naturopaths, who practice in the historical model as natural health consultants, empowering their clients with natural health information, have been pressing for passage of laws to protect their right to practice and ensure freedom of healthcare choice for consumers.

The legal wars and division in the field of naturopathy makes a case for the need for healing in healthcare. It is time for integration of healthcare practices, science and spirituality, and the old and new physics. As we shall soon see, the new physics shows us that all medicine is fundamentally energy medicine, because *everything is energy*—although the energetic effects of Western medical interventions are not necessarily health-enhancing.

The New Physics

My difficulty reconciling logic with intuition is a reflection of the left brain-right brain split in our Western culture and medical practices. The laws of Newtonian physics speak the language of the *left* hemisphere of the brain; logical and linear. In describing the behavior of subatomic particles, the laws of quantum physics speak the language of the *right* hemisphere of the brain with words like *spontaneous, connectedness, simultaneous,* and *intuitive.* One side of the brain is not "better" than the other—we need both hemispheres of our brain to work together, just as we need both branches of physics to understand the world.

In an effort to discover the ultimate building block of matter, physicists studied the physical world on a smaller and smaller scale. But what they found in this subatomic realm shattered long-held beliefs about physical reality. The substance of our world is not solid matter. It is *energy*. Quantum particles are not just composed of energy; they simply *are* energy and appear to make decisions with intelligence and consciousness.

What Newtonian physicists considered as the vacuum of space and the "nothingness" between subatomic particles is actually teeming with activity. In this quantum world, subatomic particles aren't "things," but interactions between fields of energy.

These subatomic particles spin, vibrate and produce waves as they constantly change form through a continuous process of destruction and creation that science journalist Gary Zukav likens to a dance in *The Dancing Wu Li Masters: An Overview of the New Physics*. He writes, "At the subatomic level, there is no longer a clear distinction between what is and what happens, between the actor and the action. At the subatomic level the dancer and the dance are one."

Through research experiments that have produced remarkably consistent results, quantum physicists have provided a window into a strange microscopic world that defies rational thinking and requires a cognitive leap similar to what is undertaken on the path to enlightenment. In fact, quantum physics has more in common with Eastern religions than with other branches of science. It is the bridge between Eastern and Western philosophies where imposed separations disappear—between science and spirituality, space and time, nature and self, and mind and matter. Although historically "absolute objectivity" has been the emphasis in studying science, through quantum physics we now know that objectivity is impossible and separateness is an illusion because *we cannot observe reality without altering it.*

Quantum physics greatest contribution to science may be

Bell's Theorem, published in 1964. This mathematical construct demonstrates the interdependent nature of the universe and takes quantum principles to the macro level. The inherent inseparability found in quantum phenomena on both the microscopic and macroscopic levels is compatible with the pervasive sense of unity found in enlightened states.

In quantum physics, reality is not as it appears to the Western mind. Consistent with Eastern philosophy, quantum experiments reveal physical reality as a mental construct that doesn't exist until we observe it. In our world of transient reality, information is transmitted subliminally, or faster than the speed of light, and objects, time, and space are illusionary. Through the study of quantum phenomenon, our universe is defined as a dynamic web of interconnected energy patterns where the observer's thoughts directly impact physical reality.

The old understanding of the world as mechanistic has been replaced in the scientific world but not yet in the Western mind or in Western medicine. We need a new level of understanding ourselves as beings of *energy*, because that understanding is the key to health.

Let's look at what the new physics is telling us about our body and mind, and our relationship to the world.

The New Physics and Living Beings

In her book *The Field: The Quest for the Secret Force of the Universe,* investigative journalist Lynne McTaggart details the work of scientists whose experiments have challenged the accepted Western view of life processes. Although the focus of scientific research has traditionally been about validating already accepted ideas, pioneering scientists from a wide variety of disciplines throughout the world have conducted research that applies the findings of quantum physics to living beings. Their discoveries regarding the unity between what physicists refer to as the *Zero Point Field* and all living things tells us much about the nature of health, illness, and healing, with findings that have stood up over time despite attempts to discredit them.

As often happens, what appears to be an outlandish idea will first emerge in our culture through science fiction; in books, movies, television, and more recently computer games. The concept of an underlying field of energy that connects everything in the universe—past, present and future, like "The Force" in the science fiction film *Star Wars*—is neither new nor fictional. Scientists have validated the existence of the Zero Point Field, an energetic sea that we are all part of and constantly interact with on the subatomic, molecular and cellular level. This field is the medium through which light, sound and movement travels, and all life exists.

From the ancient Greek term "ether" to more modern references such as "the divine matrix" coined by scientist, visionary and author Gregg Braden, the concept of a universal field of energy as the source of all life has been part of our consciousness for millennia.

But how was this field formed? In the "Big Bang" theory of the creation of our universe, just prior to this explosion, the entire universe was compressed into a tiny, intensely hot ball. According to this theory, everything in our universe was once physically connected in this ball, and even though the particles are now spread out over an incomprehensibly vast area, they remain always connected through the medium of the field.

In each living cell, molecules communicate through energy

in the form of wave patterns. Every molecule and every cell in the body are in constant contact with all other molecules and cells through these energetic frequencies. All body systems function in a cooperative manner orchestrated by these waves of energy that coordinate and synchronize all cellular activities. Communication occurs through wave patterns that are held in the fluid within each cell. These waves have the ability to encode information *holographically*, meaning that each piece of the encrypted information contains the whole. As every particle was once physically connected, this communication is nonlocal, or at a distance, and instantaneous.

Have you ever known something instantly, or before it even happened? The instantaneous nature of life cannot be explained by a linear flow of information between firing synapses, or chemical reactions in the body, because these processes happen far too slowly. If we are separate beings with no connection between ourselves and others, and no connection between body and mind, instant communication would not be possible. This instantaneous communication through wave resonance can be seen in the coordinated movements of a school of fish, or a flock of birds.

The driving force of the body is *energy*, not biochemistry, and as such, to be healthy is to have coherence at the quantum level. Biochemical reactions are *secondary to* and *initiated by* energy. When quantum fluctuations are disturbed and communication breaks down, when the natural emission of light in the body in the form of biophotons is blocked and the body can't self-repair, the result is illness and disease.

Naturally occurring cancer cells and pathogens in the body proliferate when quantum coherence in the body is disturbed. In naturopathic philosophy, pathogens such as viruses, bacteria, parasites, and fungi are *not* considered the primary cause of disease, but are the *result of* disruptions in our energy systems. Disturbances in our energy systems are related to physical, emotional, mental and spiritual imbalances that create an environment conducive to pathogen replication in our physical bodies. In *Philosophy of Natural Therapeutics,* Henry Lindlahr, M.D., an early founder of American naturopathy, writes "All disease is caused by something which interferes with, diminishes or disturbs the normal inflow and distribution of vital energy throughout the system."

There is no question that proliferating cancerous cells and pathogens cause suffering, illness and death, and that biochemical drugs do eradicate their presence, thereby bringing relief and saving lives. However, eliminating them with drugs is like shooting the messenger. Such treatment does not address the imbalance that caused the illness in the first place, and this is why there is a high recurrence rate of infections and cancer. Until the imbalance is corrected, health is not restored.

In quantum science the neutralizing of disorders and disease conditions in the body is accomplished through vibrational medicine—the introduction of a specific *out-of-sync* wave. When two waves are *in sync*, their peaks and troughs match up. Two waves that peak opposite of each other are said to be "out of phase," or "out of sync." When an out of sync wave is introduced into the body in the form of vibrational medicine, something remarkable happens. The wave of the targeted pathogen, cancerous cell, or toxin is in effect *canceled*. And the frequency of that target disintegrates in a process called *destructive interference*. This process restores vibrational coherence of the organism, thereby restoring health.

With the use of vibrational medicine, there are no side effects other than a "healing crisis," a temporary worsening of symptoms that can happen in the process of healing. This technology, along with energy medicine therapies that correct underlying energetic imbalances, were pivotal in facilitating the healing of my son, Jacob, from autism. In later chapters, we will be hearing more about Jacob's story as we explore vibrational medicine.

The Collective Consciousness

Another aspect of the universal energy field is the concept of a *collective consciousness*. This "information field," sometimes referred to as "hive mind," is thought to contain the collective psyche, intelligence, and wisdom of humanity. Scientists have discovered a means to explore the existence of a collective consciousness by studying how individuals and groups use intention to influence Random Event Generators, or REG machines. These REG machines, also known as "black boxes," are electronic devices designed to produce a random series of either 0s or 1s. Since the outcome of a quantum event cannot be predicted, even when past outcomes are known, the numbers produced by REGs are driven by a truly random process. Influence from the focused intention of humans registers on the REG machine as a deviation from a random 50-50 outcome.

REG machines placed around the globe in secret locations each recorded such a deviation from randomness on September 6, 1997, the day of the funeral of Diana, Princess of Wales, an event watched around the world. The REG machines recorded a similar deviation four hours *before* the planes crashed into the twin towers of the World Trade Center on September 11, 2001, suggesting that premonition is not a special ability found in only certain people, but present among all humans. Indeed, quantum physicists have discovered that transmitted information can actually arrive at its destination *before* it has even left its source.

If the collective effect of these events on the world consciousness registered on REG machines, imagine the effect of intentional influence if masses of people worked together to create specific outcomes. Researchers have discovered that the combined intent of as little as one percent of the square root of a population can create an intentional effect on that population. There are ongoing intention experiments involving groups of individuals focusing their intention toward a predetermined goal, such as reducing the crime rate in a particular city. Information on how you can become a part of these experiments can be found at www.theintentionexperiment.com.

I had my own unusual experience with the collective consciousness a few years ago, when a woman from halfway across the country contacted me because she had a dream about me. She had never met me before, never been to the state where I live, never even heard of me. Yet in the dream she was given my full name and was able to locate my contact information on the Internet. Even though I was a complete stranger to her and she had no prior experience in remote viewing or any training to enhance her intuitive abilities, from her dream she was able to accurately describe household projects I was working on at the time, as well as the inside of my house, down to the Star Wars sheets on my son's bed.

This experience showed me firsthand how intimately connected we all are through the medium of the universal energy field. The mystery lady had spontaneously accessed information about me through the collective consciousness during the right brain dominant state that occurs to all of us when we are asleep.

Healing practitioners access the universal energy field and the collective healing force during a similar right brain dominant state that occurs with the intention of helping self or others. There is physical evidence that, through their training, healing practitioners gain greater coherence, as well as greater ability to harness their own energy to create energetic order in their clients to restore quantum resonance.

Research suggests that imagination and creativity do not exist in our brains, but are an interaction with the field. To experience inspiration and intuition may simply be greater access to the field. Everyone has the potential to access all the information in the field, and as demonstrated by experiments with REG. machines, everyone is capable of premonition, intuition, and the ability to influence other living things.

A New Direction

While a tradition of energy-based healing modalities has continued uninterrupted in the East, as we have learned, the West went in a different direction in the name of science. The result has been a split from spirituality—dividing self from nature, and treating the body as a biochemical machine that operates in a fragmented, linear fashion. Ironically, it is science that has brought us full circle, back to the holistic energy-based treatments that once flourished in the U.S. and beyond—to modalities like vibrational medicine, which are therapeutic formulas that use created quantum waveforms.

With traditional methods of healing now scientifically validated, we are returning to our roots, a movement driven by the healthcare choices of millions of American consumers. We are in the midst of a medical revolution as ever-increasing numbers of

Americans vote with their wallets; choosing energy-based modalities in record numbers, and being willing to pay for them out of pocket.

Ten years ago, I got blank looks if I mentioned I practiced modalities like craniosacral therapy, Reiki, and Emotional Freedom Techniques. Today, the majority of people I encounter have some familiarity with these therapies.

For some of my clients, the question remains: all this information about energy, fields, and waveforms is all well and good, but how does it apply to me?

To answer that question, I want to introduce you to Steven, another client whose life traumas will take us to a deeper level of understanding about the role of energy in wounding... and healing.

In this chapter we have learned that everything is energy. This would include *words*. In *The Hidden Messages in Water*, Japanese researcher Dr. Masaru Emoto writes "... words themselves actually emit a unique vibration that the water is sensing. When water is shown a written word, it receives it as vibration, and expresses the message in a specific form, like a visual code for expressing words." As the human body is largely composed of water, let the energy of these word affirmations provide you with a "dose" of energy medicine.

Even though I may be feeling stuck in my life, or feel like I'm falling apart and unsure of how to proceed, at my core I know I am whole and good, and that my answers will be revealed in the right time and space.

Even though I don't trust or am afraid of my own intuition, and may have been placing a higher value on the beliefs of others over my own instincts, I am open to the possibility that we all have the ability to sense and read energy, including myself.

Even though I may feel some anxiety and resistance to concepts that are outside my accepted beliefs about life and health, I am a completely acceptable person. I take a deep breath and acknowledge that anxiety and resistance with compassion.

3

ENERGY DYNAMICS

"Everything is energy and that's all there is to it.
Match the frequency of the reality you want and you cannot
help but get that reality. It can be no other way.
This is not philosophy. This is physics."

—ALBERT EINSTEIN, PH.D.

THE FIRST TIME I MET STEVEN, a slight man in his 50s with a salt and pepper beard who came to me seeking healing for a number of issues, I noticed a frightened look in his eyes. What seemed at odds with his otherwise warm and receptive demeanor was his uneasiness, visible in the way he remained subtly on-guard. He seemed unable to relax into the chair as we spoke. It didn't take long in my initial interview to discover the source. As a young man in his 20s, Steven had been the one to find his murdered fiancé's body, and it was as if his eyes were still locked in the horror of that sight.

For the past ten years, Steven had experienced various difficulties, including problems with memory, reading comprehension, and eye-tracking—known as "visual convergence." He suffered from anxiety, headaches, "brain fog," and difficulties with processing information. Due to these processing difficulties, he had to take early retirement from a job he loved as a college professor because he no longer felt he had the "brain energy" to continue doing his job.

"Since I retired, I've been having problems with drinking and gambling. And I find myself dating one unstable woman after another. It finally dawned on me that I've gone from one addiction to another. First it was being a workaholic, now an alcoholic. On top of that I seem to be attracted to women whose lives are intense and messy. I can *see* the problems I'm causing myself with these poor choices—and yet I can't seem to do anything to stop myself. I have to get to the bottom of this," said Steven.

As Steven reclined on my healing table, I sat to his left and lightly placed one hand on his hip and the other on his shoulder. In a moment I began to sense his energy rhythms. They felt jangly and disorganized.

SESSION NOTES:

When I am working with a client and tune-in to their energy rhythms, it is like using the dial on a radio to tune in to the right frequency to hear a station. I tune in to the frequencies of my client by being in a meditative state, listening with all my senses.

With my hands resting on the client's physical body, the frequencies present to me as vibrations and waves that are unique to each individual. The vibrations can feel like a faint electrical current, a tingling sensation like the subtle humming of an electrical device. The sensations start in my hands and can spread to my whole body, often accompanied by sound and image. These waves of energy produce a corresponding color and sound that will be detailed in chapter 4.

Harmonious vibrations have a smooth feel, a pleasing sound, and look like evenly spaced rounded waves in my mind's eye.

The frequency of Steven's vibrations felt discordant with a jarring feel, a grating sound, and waves that looked spiky and irregular—a vibration pattern I have come to associate with emotions and memories that are being suppressed or kept unconscious. His frequencies felt unpleasant to me. I could only imagine what it must have been like for him.

"What do you notice in your body, Steven?" I asked.

"I feel pressure in my head, behind my eyes."

"Does this pressure have a shape? How big is it?"

"It feels round. The size of a tennis ball."

I often ask clients to describe body sensations to help them be in the moment. This is a form of mindfulness meditation which helps clients observe their thoughts, emotions and sensations in the present moment. Accepting the thought, emotion or sensation at face value is an act that is both loving and liberating.

In *Coming to Our Senses: Healing Ourselves and the World through Mindfulness*, scientist and meditation teacher Jon Kabat-Zinn describes mindfulness meditation—"It is really an inward gesture that inclines the heart and mind (seen as one seamless whole) toward a full-spectrum awareness of the present moment just as it is, accepting whatever is happening simply because it is already happening."

"Does the area of pressure behind your eyes have a color?" I asked Steven.

"Black," he replied.

I recalled what William Redpath, psychoanalyst, certified advanced Rolfer, and author of *Trauma Energetics: A Study of Held-Energy Systems* wrote about the relationship between colors and subtle energies. In Redpath's extensive experience, areas in the body sensed as black lack vibration and energetic movement. These perceived areas of blackness are both the key to locating the body areas where trauma can be accessed, and the key to releasing them.

Redpath discovered that focusing on color and shape initiates access to "held-energy systems," or areas where trauma has created arrested energy flow. It is important to focus on the attributes of the held energy area, rather than the traumatic memory itself, in order to prevent retraumatization. Reliving the memory can in itself become another traumatic event.

I advised Stephen, "Just allow this tennis-ball-sized area of black tension to express in whatever way it needs to while you focus your attention on it and send your breath into it."

"You know, I just realized this is the same area where my headache starts, and where that brain fog feeling comes from," Steven added.

"That's a good observation. Notice those thoughts while you stay focused on the tension. Allow yourself to drop into the area behind your eyes with your awareness," I suggested.

This is a basic step in the healing process—helping the client learn how to "step outside themselves." Doing so helps us become more acutely self-aware of feelings, symptoms, and how the body reacts to certain people and situations. By avoiding any attempt to dictate or control the process, we in essence "get out of the way" of our own healing.

"I'm trying to make the black change to light," Steven continued.

"It's best to just *hang out* with the tension and not try to change it," I responded. "The more you can allow it to just *be* and let go of any expectation that it move, the more you allow the healing process to unfold."

Steven's desire to manage his healing process is understandable. In our everyday lives, the ability to effect change and control outcomes through *force* is a common, even desired drive, especially when we are in fear.

"But how do I 'let go'?" Stephen asked. "I've tried to fight this thing. And I've tried to ignore it. It's a terrible feeling. If I let go, I feel like I'll just fall apart, or lose my mind."

This is an almost universal fear—the fear of losing control. Letting go doesn't feel safe because we don't trust, but I have found that attempts to direct the healing process only serve to keep the area of held energy in an arrested pattern, until it is faced unconditionally. *Allowing* the healing process to proceed without interference is an act of respect and acceptance that creates a sense of trust critical to the release process. We will be revisiting this vital concept in later chapters.

As Steven joined me in witnessing his tension pattern, I was able to sense with my hands that his energy was working with mine to facilitate his healing. At once, the energy flow to the area of tension increased. Steven had willfully entered into his healing process.

I can also sense when a client is losing focus. In that case, their energy will suddenly feel absent from the process, which tells me they are no longer engaged. By simply asking them what they notice about the sensation we are working with, they quickly become refocused and reengaged.

Before we continue with Steven's story, it's important to talk more about what it means to be the observer, or the witness, and the distinction between interfering and creating.

The New Physics Revisited

From the science of quantum physics we know that one cannot observe reality without changing it. In other words, to *observe* is to *participate*. Scientists have found that the act of looking at a subatomic particle changes the particle's behavior in the moment that we are looking at it. As everything is made of subatomic particles, including us, in witnessing ourselves we have the opportunity to participate in ultimate reality and to make a *choice*. To become a participant in our healing process, we have only to observe *without* conditions.

The moment that Steven and I became focused on his area of tension, the particles began to respond by pulsing, a sensation one might experience immediately after an injury when blood flow and energy are rushing to the area. I have found that this pulsing sensation precedes the release of tension and the resumption of energy flow.

Another important aspect of observing is our state of mind as we observe. In 1927, quantum physicists Niels Bohr and Werner Heisenberg discovered the nature of the universe as an infinite number of possibilities that exist simultaneously. This would include the possibility of complete healing. In effect, our thoughts and feelings select which possibility becomes reality. I see my client as already healed and *feel* what it would be like for them to be completely healed, and suggest they do the same. The act of choosing the possibility of healing with your thoughts and feelings, while being *detached* from the outcome and the *details* of how and when that healing will occur, is an act of creation.

This combination of observing an issue in a state of accepting it as it is—while choosing which possibility you desire with your thoughts and feelings in a detached state—is the key to creating your life. Now when I talk about detachment, I don't mean suppressing your feelings and pretending you don't care. It's about *feeling* your feelings, and then letting go. We will be revisiting these important concepts in later chapters.

As I worked with Steven, a large amount of information about the nature of his issue came to my mind in a single instant. When this happens spontaneously, I know I have connected to the universal field of energy and "downloaded" information, similar to the way one would download a picture or document from "cyberspace" to your computer. But unlike a computer, this downloaded information is received through a shift in consciousness rather than reaching for something outside of ourselves, which implies a separation that does not exist. Both the information and ourselves are part of the field.

Now I need to digress here, to help you understand this "information download" that can happen during an energy healing session. Because it happens in a split-second of time, allow me to slow it down for you, and help you understand it as well.

Information in an Instant

As Steven's session continued, my mind began to scan through the information that I had received in that instant, like scrolling through a downloaded file. It can take me an hour or more to process through all the information that comes more or less "holographically." By that I mean, the single piece contains the whole—or to say it another way, the download contains both image and the far-ranging effects of the incident or incidents depicted, all in one sudden flash.

Intuitives of all types will recognize these occurrences. For example, author and professional writing consultant David Hazard explains his experience this way:

"A writer will begin to explain the book they're writing to me, but instead of focusing on their words I focus 'beyond them'—waiting to see if what I call 'a greater concept' will present itself to me *through* their words. In short, I stay open. Sometimes nothing happens, and in those cases I advise them how to proceed with their writing based on the ideas they've told me. It's very cut-and-dried. But many times a whole new concept will more or less *explode* in front of my mind's-eye. I 'get' the whole book— title, cover design, chapters, everything—in a split-second. It's like reading the whole book that they are *meant* to write, when they don't even know about it yet. And it can take me an hour or more to describe and explain the presentation and content to them."

"When I tell them the concept, they're stunned. 'That *is* it. It's like the idea was stuck inside me and I didn't even know it was there.'

"When I've explained this to a few friends who are also in publishing they've said, 'This happens because you've been working with writers for so many years.' But that's not the case. They're not the result of experience or training—though I've now trained myself how to get in a mentally open frame of mind where these experiences can occur. The truth is these experiences have happened to me from the time I was a junior-level editor. They come from someplace that's outside of formal training."

Not surprisingly, David has practiced meditation for nearly 30 years, and honed his ability to focus his attention and be present to himself and other people.

As David's writing student described, it seemed as if he had accessed a book idea that was inside of them. But if that were true, where would that idea be located? And more importantly, how could David access information that was located inside someone else's mind?

I used to believe that the memory of traumatic events was located in our brains and held in the cells and tissues impacted by the trauma. But if that were so, then how was it possible that I could see someone else's memory in my own mind, and feel their trauma in my own body? The findings of research scientists shed some light on these puzzling questions.

Neurosurgeon and research scientist Karl Pribram discovered that, even after destroying virtually every part of a rat's brain, the rat still remembered a previously learned routine. If the memory of a routine was not stored in the rat's brain, then where was it? We now know that the brain does not *store* information; it is the *receiver* and *processer* of information, and that ability to receive and process is distributed throughout the brain. Research suggests that memory is not located in the body at all, but in the universal energy field, making up the collective consciousness that we all have access to.

Based on my experiences with clients, I now believe that the receptors on the surface of every cell in the body function as receivers of memory, rather than storing the memory itself. When we direct our attention to traumatized body tissues in an observing and allowing state of mind, we gain access to information about that trauma through our energy systems, from the universal energy field. As we are all connected through the medium of the universal energy field, this is how I am able to see, feel, and hear information that is not part of my personal experience.

So, where does information about a writer's unformed

thoughts, or the true source of a client's wounds or illness lie?

The Field

Although the Western scientific community dismisses the possibility of accessing information in this manner, the C.I.A. took it seriously enough to conduct successful programs in "remote viewing," that is, obtaining information from a distance by connecting with the universal energy field. These C.I.A. programs are detailed in science journalist Lynne McTaggart's book *The Field*.

Getting back to Pribram's research, we can see how his findings have implications for the nature of sight as well. We do not see by projecting an image onto the brain or on our retinas, as is commonly accepted. Rather, we receive information from images in the form of wave patterns. The lens of the eye converts these waves into virtual images, similar to how a laser hologram works. Both seeing and memory are about accessing the field, and interpreting the energy waves that are encoded with information.

Here's what's important for you to know about tapping into these information downloads.

Possessing an ability to access the field and retrieve information is not a special gift that only certain people have. I am not "special" because I've learned to do this. Everyone has this ability, just as anyone has the ability, for instance, to learn to play the piano. If you put years of intention and practice into it, you could become a concert pianist. But even without piano training, almost anyone can manage to play "Chopsticks."

Drawing again from the computer analogy, the more one upgrades their "operating system" through healing, the faster and more efficiently they can "download" information from the universal energy field. And with those upgrades comes the capability of downloading more complex "files" that contain audio, video, and even "special effects."After many years of developing this ability through personal growth facilitated by classes, practice, and restoring the flow of my own energy with the help of healing therapists, I access the field by being in a mindful meditative state. Shifting into a right brain dominant state initiates the unfolding of the process of healing.

When I began my own healing process in 1992, it was as if I were operating at a level of "Heidi 1.0." Negative thoughts would frequently interfere with my ability to stay in the moment; self-critical and self-doubting thoughts that got in the way of my ability to access the field for intuition. But after years of training, experience, and personal growth; it is as if I have upgraded to a new operating system many times over—now functioning on a level of say, "Heidi 10.0!" And this more highly evolved operating system is required for me to run a healing therapist "program."

Now I want to tell you about the information itself.

The information received from the field can contain visual images and auditory information with words describing the situation I am viewing, as if I am playing back a narrated video. The information can also contain physical and emotional information, where I feel what the client feels in the scene, both emotional and physical sensations such as pain or tightness in specific areas of my body. As long as I maintain my separateness even while being connected to my client, it is clear that these emotions and sensations are not mine. I have on occasion taken on a client's "stuff," especially in the early years of my practice, but when these situations arise, I view them as helpful indicators of where my own system needs additional work.

The downloaded information can also include scenes that

contain images that would not be possible in everyday life, like you might see in a film with computer generated imagery (CGI) or 3D computer graphics, such as seeing the flow of energy as streamers of colored light, or seeing inside someone's body.

Occasionally I continue to perceive information about a client's situation *after* the session has ended because I am unable to process through all the information, images, symbols, and metaphors that came through in an instant *during* the session. Or sometimes I am only able to interpret one part of the information, and I get the bigger picture later. For example, Brooke came to me with a complex health history of several serious and debilitating autoimmune diseases that began after a car accident nine years earlier. The extent of disability in a young person following an accident that caused no harm to other passengers baffled her Western medical doctors.

During Brooke's session, I had a sudden flash of information that contained words and pictures showing me where the force of the accident had entered her body and disrupted her energy systems, and how that force was still active in her systems, as well as how to best help her. However, it wasn't until later that evening after the session was over that I had a sudden *knowing* of how even earlier trauma had weakened Brooke's energy systems, leaving her vulnerable to the cascading symptoms and illnesses that began after the auto accident. In these instances, I suddenly *know* things about a client's situation that I didn't know the moment before. And I have to interpret this "knowing" into language and may not be able to make sense of all of the information to relate it to the client until a later session.

Before we return to Steven, it is important to tell you what scientists have discovered about healing practitioners.

Working with The Field

In *Energy Medicine: The Scientific Basis*, cellular biologist and physiologist James Oschman details the findings of medical researchers, including the discovery that the biomagnetic field of healing practitioners extends *into* the energy field and physical body of the healing client during a healing session. An unusually high energy field pattern has been documented around healing practitioners during healing sessions and a strong biomagnetic field has been recorded radiating from a healing practitioner's hands while they are in a meditative state. The field of energy emitted from healing practitioners has been found to fluctuate through a wide range of frequencies known to activate healing in a variety of hard and soft tissues, naturally communicating the necessary signals for cell repair.

Man-made instruments, such as pulsed electromagnetic field (PEMF) therapy devices used by physicians to "jump start" healing in bone fractures that have failed to heal, as well as ultrasound therapy and low level laser therapy cannot engage in two-way communication and adjust frequencies accordingly, the way living systems can. These instruments can only emit the frequency to which they are set. Human hands can emit more than one frequency at a time when more than one intention is used. Oschman hypothesizes, "...no medical device, regardless of its sophistication, is likely to achieve the efficacy and safety obtainable by imposing a naturally generated signal to living tissue."

With years of practicing hands-on healing, healing practitioners would be expected to have brain changes similar to those documented in musicians in areas of the brain involved in their work. In a study of string instrument players, brain areas that controlled movement and sensation of the fingers used in playing their instrument increased in size and produced more intense brain waves and biomagnetic fields. The more years the musician had practiced their instrument, the more pronounced were these naturally produced brain modifications. This is consistent with the growing body of research from the field of neuroplasticity presented in *Train Your Mind, Change Your Brain: How a New Science Reveals Our Extraordinary Potential to Transform Ourselves,* by science writer Sharon Begley.

Research on brain plasticity strikes a blow to the Western belief that adult brains are unchangeable and our behaviors are determined by genes and neurotransmitters. Scientific studies indicate that the way we live our lives actually shapes our brains. Using neural stem cells, the brain is capable of growing new neurons throughout the lifespan.

When signals are cut from a body part to the brain, the corresponding part of the brain does not atrophy. Rather, it can begin processing signals for a completely different body part. For example, the visual cortex is capable of processing hearing in a person who becomes blind and the auditory cortex can begin processing visual input for a deaf person. The visual and auditory cortexes can even assume the jobs of feeling and processing language.

The implications of neuroplasticity research for healing are staggering. We are not doomed to a life dictated by our genes, with no possibility of changing how our brains became wired during childhood. Through the study of individuals with obsessive compulsive disorder and depression, researchers have discovered that by simply having the research subjects practice observing their thoughts as *events*, rather than allowing the thoughts to become their *identity,* both brain chemistry and brain circuit activity was altered, resulting in a significant reduction in symptoms and rate of relapse. A study of experienced mindfulness meditators revealed unusually high gamma brain wave patterns during meditation and an elevated gamma wave baseline when they weren't meditating, indicating mindfulness creates enduring brain changes.

In experiments conducted specifically on healing practitioners from a wide variety of healing disciplines, physicist Robert C. Beck studied how their brains reacted as they practiced their healing methods. Regardless of which healing modality they practiced, while actively engaged in their work the healing practitioners' brain waves were recorded in a range consistent with altered states of consciousness. He also discovered that their brain waves became synchronized with the Earth's geomagnetic field while occupied in healing activities. This synchronization of wave frequencies to the same rhythm is known in physics as entrainment.

When a healing practitioner lays their hands on a client, they are not just touching the skin. Due to the interconnected nature of the body, their touch actually extends through what Oschman refers to as "the living matrix," a fully integrated network that facilitates mechanical, electrical, and energetic information exchange. In other words, the skin is connected to underlying connective tissue, which in turn is intimately joined to the very interior of each cell in a remarkable continuity that involves literally every molecule of the body.

The Release of Immobilized Energy

Returning to Steven and what was happening as he lay there on my table, with our combined energies coursing through the area of his brain that needed healing, we can now look at the accessed information that told me *how* he needed to heal.

With my hands becoming very warm from the flow of energy

as I cradled Steven's skull, my mind began to scan through the information I had accessed from the field. A scene began to play of Steven as a young man as he discovered that his fiancé had been murdered. I was shown how at the moment he saw her bludgeoned body, the trauma of the event was taken in through his eyes. The scene included images that showed me how the flow of energy behind his eyes became immobilized. The energy became "frozen," similar to the way an animal who feels threatened will "play dead."

These images are consistent with Redpath's discovery that the energy effects of trauma become established in the body instantaneously. The body can maintain and isolate these effects from energy flow for years, but doing so requires a lot of energy. According to Redpath, the brain scans an area of immobilized energy approximately ten times per second. But just as the trauma effects were set in place instantly, the arrested energy can be restored to movement just as quickly, regardless of how long it has been in this holding pattern.

As Steven and I worked with the pulsing area behind his eyes, the area of tension the size of a tennis ball that he initially described began to change to a more diffuse area that to his senses had the consistency of molasses. And then Steven began to fidget.

"Are you feeling uncomfortable?" I asked.

"Yes. I feel like I have to move my arms and legs around. I just can't seem to get comfortable."

Fidgeting is a common response I see during a healing session just prior to the release experience. It is an unconscious attempt on the part of the client to relieve the tension created when connecting with emotions by moving the body.

"And my bladder is full," continued Steven. "Which is

strange, because I just emptied it before we started." This natural *diuretic* effect, a temporary increase in the rate of urination, occurs due to the detoxifying action of energy medicine, the removal of toxins from the physical, subtle, emotional, mental, and spiritual bodies. In fact, my clients sometimes have to empty their bladder before, during, and after an energy healing session.

Now here's the part that may sound strange. The area of tension Steven and I were focusing on began to *move* around in his body.

As I am working with an area of arrested energy flow, the sensation of pain, pressure, or tension will often suddenly change location. When we focus on an area of immobilized energy, we are engaging it on an energetic level, which makes it more difficult for the body to keep the area isolated from energy circulation. Just as we focus on it, the location of the sensation can inexplicably move, as if trying to "throw us off"—the body reacts to our focus by attempting to draw our attention away from the area. It seems to not want to be seen, as being seen interferes with its ability to keep the area encapsulated. The body-mind is simply doing its job of protection by keeping painful emotions suppressed and hidden. When the sensation moves in this manner, I take it as an encouraging sign that we've "blown its cover."

John Sarno, M.D., an expert in musculoskeletal pain, theorizes that the role of pain is to keep emotions suppressed below the level of consciousness, because physical pain is more acceptable in our society than emotional pain. This theory rings true in my work as a healing therapist. Sensations of pain, tension and pressure will often present the moment a client lays on the healing table, in the therapeutic presence of unconditional acceptance. The client may be baffled by these sensations, unable to recall any physical event that would account for this discomfort that wasn't even in their awareness until that moment. The sudden appearance of pain and pressure are not indicative of an injury, but of the presence of suppressed emotions.

As long as the client continues to breathe into the area where the tension *first* appeared, what I call "ground zero," while letting go of trying to change it and allowing the tension pattern to fully express in whatever manner it needs to, the tension will eventually release. The more fully one is able to surrender and let go, the more quickly the immobilized energy will resume flowing.

Steven's trauma had left him with arrested energy flow in the area behind his eyes for three decades, where body, mind and spirit remained immobilized, disturbing the flow of biological communication required for cell repair. Eventually, this ongoing state gave rise to Steven's symptoms—the visual difficulties and headaches. As arrested energy flow creates a sensation of heaviness and a feeling of being stuck and disconnected, release and restoration of energy flow creates a sensation of movement and a feeling of lightness as the flow of blood, oxygen, and biological substrates are restored.

As the tension in Steven's head began to dissipate, I detected a softening, expansive sensation in my hands. Steven described how the black had changed to red, and then to light, accompanied by a feeling of lightness. With the release of the long-held energy of his trauma, Steven's whole body started to shake, and he began to cry.

The shaking I observed in Steven is a result of the human physiological reaction to perceived danger—a basic mammalian response. Mammals react to perceived danger with a "fight or flight" response, initiated by energy. This response encompasses the rapid mobilization of the sympathetic nervous system and the neuroendocrine system with a release of stress hormones into the bloodstream. If the animal is unable to escape, the protective response of the parasympathetic system through neurohormone release causes it to collapse. In this collapsed state, the animal is disassociated from its body, physically frozen and in shock. Until the danger passes, the sympathetic response remains active, even while the animal is in this dissociative, frozen state. Once the danger has passed, the energy charge initiated by the dangerous situation is released through full-body shaking.

If this entire process—the energy-initiated hormone response, the dissociative state, and the release of the charge—occurs without interruption, no trauma is produced. However, if natural recovery is blocked, which can occur if the danger does not pass or the energy discharge does not occur, trauma occurs and the energy charge remains active in energy systems for weeks, months, years, or even a lifetime, exacting a huge toll on our health. Psycho-physiological trauma theorist Paul Levine, Ph.D., author of *Waking the Tiger: Healing Trauma,* refers to this state as "shock traumatization."

You may have had this experience of shaking after a close call from a dangerous situation, such as narrowly averting a car accident. Once the danger passed, you may have begun trembling all over. Now what would happen if that sense of danger never passed, or your trembling response was blocked and suppressed? In healing scenarios, completing the "trauma circle" occurs when we finally have that energy discharge, perhaps many years after the initial traumatic incident. It occurs when we feel *safe.*

Once a sense of safety has been achieved, such as during a healing session with a trusted therapist, this nervous system charge naturally diffuses. In a healing session, the shaking that results is usually obvious, but sometimes clients indicate they have a "feeling" of internal shaking that is not externally visible. For a number of my clients, the sense of safety achieved during the session may be happening for the first time in their life.

A Word about "Stress"

So we see that the sense of danger must pass before full recovery from trauma can take place. But for some, that never happens. You may recognize this pervasive sense of unease that negatively affects your health as *stress*.

What exactly is stress? Stress is an umbrella term used to define our response to anything perceived as a threat to well-being. This would include "stressful" events such as public speaking, changing jobs, or an impending deadline. When these pressure, fear, and worry-filled situations disrupt energy, the sympathetic nervous system mobilizes in response, producing the physical, emotional, mental, and spiritually distressing sensations we refer to as "feeling stressed." These sensations can include headaches, body tension, upset stomach, and feeling anxious, overwhelmed and isolated. But the bigger question is—why do we respond to these situations as threats to our well-being? Why does one person feel stress in response to, for example, public speaking, while another does not?

Whether or not a situation disrupts energy and triggers a sympathetic nervous system response depends on whether there is past trauma that created negative unconscious beliefs. In other words, if you have had past traumatic experiences that created a belief that standing in front of an audience and speaking is something to be feared, healing begins with becoming aware of the underlying beliefs, not through eliminating all public speaking in your life just to avoid stress.

Some of my clients whose health issues haven't responded to Western medicine have been instructed by physicians to remove all stress from their lives with the implication that once these exterior sources of stress are eliminated, their health problems will resolve. This recommendation is an example of the "outside-in" mentality of Western medicine. As we will discuss in later chapters, true healing occurs from the "inside-out."

Eliminating excess stress from one's life is an excellent goal that likely will improve one's health in the short term. However, if we avoid all situations that create stress, we can actually create stagnation and limitation by eliminating the opportunity for growth and transformation—the goal of healing. This is why it is more important to look "inside" at *why* these situations are creating stress, or why we may be intentionally creating stress in our lives by taking on too much. In that way, what is unconscious can become conscious, and we can then attend to the underlying trauma and related belief that is causing the stress response. We will be exploring beliefs that create stress and the process of healing them in later chapters.

Getting back to Steven, the energy that had been frozen in place for so long could finally complete its movement, just as an animal who has played dead will resume its normal activities once the threat has passed.

"What do you notice about the tension, Steven?" I asked.

"It's gone," he said with a furrowed brow.

"Is it OK that it's gone?" I asked.

"I've never had such severe pressure and tension just disappear like that. It makes me feel like it wasn't real. Like the problem was all in my head, no pun intended. I mean, I remember finding my fiancé's body, clear as a bell. But I don't feel any angst about it. How is that possible?"

Steven's confusion is understandable. It can be an unsettling experience to have sensations move around your body, and then disappear in an instant, and memories that have been traumatic for years suddenly lose their "charge." I assured him that the emotions he had been feeling were very real, as were his pressure and discomfort, the result of reduced oxygen supply to muscles, ligaments, tendons or nerves caused by the autonomic nerve response.

We all know how painful a heart attack is, when the heart muscle is deprived of oxygen from a blocked artery. The pain and discomfort caused by a less dramatic disruption in oxygen is just as real. This is why both the application of heat and use of "trigger point therapy," or brief manual compression, can relieve pain and tension. Both enhance oxygen flow to the affected area. However, unless the underlying cause of the tension is addressed, the relief obtained from heat and trigger point compression may only be temporary.

Although Steven's release happened in an instant, it took him most of the session to get to that moment of surrender that precedes release, as he had no frame of reference for being in that state. Clients typically experience subsequent releases much more quickly as they gain experience with the healing release process.

Once Steven was assured of the validity of his experience, he looked forward to continuing his process. After several sessions using a variety of techniques to heal his past traumas, Steven's headaches disappeared, along with his difficulties with reading comprehension, memory, and eye tracking. And although he retained his traumatic memories, the memories were neutralized.

Instead of looking frightened, Steven's eyes began to radiate his sense of joy as balance returned to his life. Once the immobilized energy from the traumas of his life was released, the anxiety that Steven had quelled with alcohol, gambling, and unstable relationships was gone. In later sessions, other blockages and disturbances in his energy would emerge, in different forms and in different energy systems. As they released, Steven's addictions, compulsions and obsessions were replaced by a sense of peace, and excitement about a future of his own creation.

In the next chapter we will look at energetic anatomy, where these blockages and disturbances occur.

Even though my impulse may be to push away undesirable thoughts, emotions, or bodily tension, I am acceptable just as I am, and I'm beginning to understand the importance of allowing my thoughts, emotions, and bodily tensions to express so that I may receive their message.

Even though I may recognize that I often get in my own way, I am learning to accept myself without conditions.

Even though I may have a fear of letting go, I am fully acceptable, and I am willing to learn more about the surrender process.

— 4 —

ENERGETIC ANATOMY

*"Many therapists who work daily and successfully with human
energy systems have felt alienated from the sciences that provide
the logical and rational foundation for conventional medicine.
A close look at energy medicine resolves this unnecessary
confusion and controversy."*

—JAMES OSCHMAN, PH.D.

I GREW UP IN A HOUSEHOLD where it was not uncommon for my mother to have "gut" feelings about people and
situations, known as *clairsentience,* and "knowing" about
circumstances, people and places without having prior knowledge, referred to as *claircognizance.* My mother once abruptly
canceled plans for a weekend trip due to an ominous feeling
she had about driving to our destination. Because these intuitive experiences were acceptable in my family of origin, I in
turn was tuned in to my own gut feelings and premonitions.

As a teenager, I had a knowing that I would marry young and

have fertility issues. But other forms of intuition were not part of my childhood environment. *Clairvoyance,* an inner seeing beyond ordinary perception, and *clairaudience,* hearing voices, music or sounds that have no physical source, were not part of the culture in which I was raised, nor were the energy systems of the body that can be perceived by using these intuitive senses, or healing techniques to work with them. When presented with information about energy systems for the first time in nursing school, it is little wonder that I strongly resisted.

You may have had similar experiences that provided you with some frame of reference for perceiving the energy systems of the body, or you may not because this information is generally not part of our education in the West, either in our schools or in our homes. But the truth is, energy systems are part of the human anatomy. In the West, we weren't taught how to recognize and understand them, much less how to work with them.

Because of this lack of knowledge about energy systems, we have impoverished ourselves when it comes to healing modalities. We do not even know the true nature of our bodies or that healing modalities exist that address disruptions in our energy bodies. As a result, many of us suffer when our energy systems are blocked or damaged without having any understanding of this vital part of our bodies. We need to restore this knowledge to live healthier, fuller lives.

In the previous chapter, I introduced the concept of energy blockages as we looked at Steven's situation. Before we can begin to explore *how* energy blockages are formed, we need to have an understanding of *where* these blockages form—in human energy systems. To assist you in this understanding, a summary of available information follows. For more detailed information on the energy systems of the body, I encourage you to consult the books that will be referenced throughout this chapter and listed in the appendix.

The Anatomy of Energy Systems

Although only a fraction of the wisdom amassed by ancient peoples regarding energy systems survived the conquering of great civilizations that preceded the Dark Ages, references to energy systems can still be found in cultures from all corners of the planet. In the illustrated *The Subtle Body: An Encyclopedia of Your Energetic Anatomy*, energy medicine therapist Cyndi Dale thoroughly explores energy systems from cultures around the world, including Chinese, Hindu, Thai, Tibetan, Cherokee, Mayan, Incan, Egyptian, and African energy systems.

Ancient civilizations developed methods for working with energy systems for the same reason I studied energy medicine, because approaching healthcare in the context of the body as energy is *effective.* Surviving theories about energy systems varies among these ancient cultures, but commonalities exist. All recognized energy as the essence of *life,* the connection between the state of that energy and *health,* and how through these systems of energy we create *reality.*

As discussed in chapter 2, our Western culture has experienced a much more recent disruption in the continuity of information when knowledge of energy and healing was largely lost following the publication of the Flexner Report in 1910. For Westerners, this resulted in a loss of understanding the intrinsic nature of our bodies as energy, and its energetic structures. Consequently, information about energy systems is not a part of our "ordinary reality." When studied in the West, energy systems are generally referred to as "non-ordinary reality," given that their existence is outside of our usually accepted view of reality.

In addition to surviving information from ancient Eastern traditions, scientific studies of the last century and the observations and experiences of modern day energy medicine practitioners—such as Barbara Brennan, Rosalyn Bruyere, and Donna Eden—have added greatly to our understanding of human energy systems. These studies and observations will be presented throughout this chapter.

For the purposes of learning about energy blockages, I will focus on the most commonly known energy systems: the human energy *field* that surrounds and permeates the physical body, oriented to a central axis; the energy *centers* that emanate from the midline of the body, known as the chakras; and the energy *channels* that run throughout the body, known as the meridians.

The Human Energy Field

As quantum physicists have established, everything is energy, including our thoughts, our beliefs, our emotions, and our bodies. The density of energy is determined by the frequency at which it vibrates. The energy of our physical bodies vibrates at a slower rate, creating matter that is dense enough to be seen with our eyes and touched with our hands. The energy of the human energy field, known as the *subtle body*, or *aura* in religious traditions, vibrates at a rate faster than the speed of light, creating a body that can only be perceived with our intuitive senses.

All living things, including plants and animals, are surrounded by a field of energy which exists within the universal energy field. *The Secret Life of Plants: A Fascinating Account of the Physical, Emotional, and Spiritual Relations Between Plants and Man,* by science journalists Peter Tompkins and Christopher Bird, is filled with research documenting the energetic nature of plants, and how they interact with humans and animals through the medium of the universal field.

For example, researchers using instruments such as the galvanometer, commonly known as a polygraph lie detector, have measured changes in electrical charge associated with thoughts and emotions. Through studies conducted by connecting plants to a galvanometer, researchers have established that plants respond to our intentions and state of emotion. This phenomenon occurs regardless of the distance the human subject is from the plant, and regardless of whether measurements are taken from an intact plant, or just a severed piece of the plant. In addition, energy fields have even been detected around inanimate objects if they were touched by a living thing.

In this chapter, when I use the phrase "the field," I am referring to the energy field around the body, which is distinct from, though exists within, the universal energy field. This field is composed of the combined fields produced by all cells and body organs, as well as the chakras, meridians and other energy structures of the body. Scientists have documented the fields related to the electrical activity of the heart and brain, and the electromagnetic properties of the human energy field that give it both repelling and attracting qualities.

We know there is an energy field in and around us and there are ways to detect it. Let's take a closer look at what it is and how it works in you.

Characteristics of the Human Energy Field

From what is known and understood about the human energy field through information from ancient civilizations, coupled with the observations of those who work in energy medicine and information from scientific studies, we know that this field is organized around a central axis between two poles, in the same way that the Earth's geomagnetic field is organized.

In the human body, the superior pole, which approximates the North Pole of the Earth, is located in the sphenoid, a bone of the cranium, or skull. The inferior pole, which approximates the South Pole of the Earth, is located in the sacrum, or tailbone. Energy flows between these two poles through the central axis, an energy pulsation that reverberates throughout the entire physical and energetic body. (see figure 4-1)

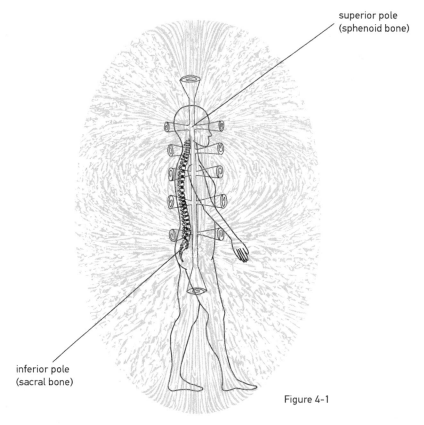

superior pole
(sphenoid bone)

inferior pole
(sacral bone)

Figure 4-1

The field is an egg-shaped container for your energy, made up of layers, and functions as a receiver and filter of energies. The most commonly accepted system of quantifying this field identifies seven layers, with the first layer near the skin and the outermost edge of the seventh layer extending several feet from the body. This field is akin to one's "personal space," the zone around us that we consider psychologically ours and which is, in fact, a part of our bodies. When two people are closer than an arm's length apart, their subtle bodies encounter each other, resulting in intimate contact that can create discomfort if unwanted.

For over a century, attempts have been made to document the human energy field through various imaging processes. The most widely-known and successful of these early attempts is Kirlian photography, invented by Russian scientist Semyon Kirlian. In 1939, Kirlian discovered that by placing living tissue on a photographic plate charged with electricity, the elicited electrical corona could be captured on film. Kirlian recognized the value of his photographic technique while conducting experiments that included himself as a research subject. Shortly after a photograph of his fingertip taken with his technique lacked a corona, he developed the flu. His wife, Valentina, also experienced the same sequence of events. Based on Kirlian's findings, which have been corroborated by further study and observation, we know that illness and disease states are *preceded by* an imbalance in the subtle body, resulting in diminished energy flow, *followed by* appearance of illness symptoms in the physical body.

The value of Kirlian photography wasn't recognized by mainstream science until the 1960s, but it has since found widespread applications in the human, animal, and plant worlds. For example, Kirlian photographs of seeds have been used in determining viability; photos of fish scales have been used in determining areas of water pollution; and photos of fingertips and human cells have been found useful in the diagnosis of disease. In one study involving 6,000 industrial workers in Romania, Kirlian photography was more effective in detecting the presence of cancer than conventional testing.

In the 1970s, experiments using Kirlian photography conducted by UCLA psychologist Dr. Thelma Moss documented the highly dynamic nature of the human energy field. Dr. Moss recorded the changes in size, shape, color, and quality of the field in response to state of health, thoughts, mood, and relationships. Kirlian photography has also documented the contraction of the field that occurs during periods of stress, illness, and depression, and expansion of the field that occurs with health, happiness, and after a healing.

During one of my first healing sessions as a practitioner, the client's energy field expanded so greatly I could no longer detect the edges within the confines of my treatment room. Having no frame of reference for this effect, I feared that I had "exploded" her energy! In time I learned that the field expands with every effective healing, to varying degrees.

Healing practitioner Rosalyn Bruyere, who has been tested off the charts on energy-measuring equipment, notes the cultural differences she has observed in the function and appearance of human energy systems in peoples around the world in her book *Wheels of Light: Chakras, Auras, and the Healing Energy of the Body.* In her experience, the energy fields of Westerners consistently differ from those she perceived around people in the Middle East. These dissimilarities are a reflection of our cultural thought processes and beliefs, and speak to the difficulty we in the West have in grasping what is innate in the East. In the West, people typically operate on the mental level and are "all in their heads," energetically disconnected from their legs and lower parts of their physical body.

When I first visited a healing therapist for my own healing, I became aware of how my energy field was "top heavy." Later, when I began working with healing clients myself, I thought it was a coincidence that each person that came through my office door had the same energy field pattern that I initially had. Over time I realized I was observing a widespread cultural phenomenon. The vast majority of clients I've worked with over the last fifteen years, especially if they've never had energy work before, have an energy field that is wide at the top, and narrow at the bottom, like the shape of the letter "V," as opposed to the oval egg-shape seen in a healthy, balanced aura.

Exploring the Human Energy Field

From the moment a healing therapist laid her hands on me, I knew in my heart that I was meant to study energy medicine and do the same work. But I put that thought aside for years while attending to my own healing. I was waiting for the "right" time, when I would be "done" with my healing process, presumably after the infertility issue was resolved. It is clear to me now that my resistance was coming from the blockages in my energy systems, but truth be told, the postponement was also related to concern about what others might think, particularly the nurses I worked with. Ironically, it was a flier posted on the unit where I worked that broke through the resistance.

My employer sponsored a one-day workshop on therapeutic touch, an energy-based healing modality developed by Dolores

Krieger, Ph.D., R.N., author of *The Therapeutic Touch: How to Use Your Hands to Help or to Heal*. The sponsorship of the workshop by the hospital neutralized my concerns about criticism in the workplace.

As the resistance began to recede, I realized that if I waited until everything in my life was complete I would never move forward, because life is an unfolding process, a series of endings and beginnings marked by growth. I could no longer keep my life on hold waiting for a baby who might never arrive.

Even after listening to the information presented at the workshop, I did not automatically accept the existence of the human energy field. I wanted to confirm its presence for myself by learning how to detect it.

One of my first explorations of the human energy field involved the use of a dowsing tool. Ancient civilizations used these tools to detect energetic frequencies. Scientists have determined that dowsers can pick up frequencies from the universal energy field through sensors that are primarily located in the solar plexus, which correlates with the expression "gut feeling." Other minor sensors for reading frequencies are located in the brain. These frequencies are amplified by the fluid in our bodies and read through the movement of the dowsing tool as it is held in the dowser's hand.

I was taught how to make dowsing rods to detect the field in that first workshop on therapeutic touch at the hospital, and came home to try it out for myself. I made a set of dowsing rods by cutting the hook off a wire hanger, cutting the remainder in half, and bending each half into an "L" shape. After slipping an appropriate length of cut drinking straw over the shorter end of each rod, I held the straws with my fingers with the long end of the wire rods extending out in front of me, several inches apart. The rods moved freely within the straws as I sought to keep them as level as possible.

Slowly walking toward a seated and open-minded friend with my homemade dowsing rods, I hoped to detect her energy field. About three feet from my friend's body, the rods suddenly swung inward and toward each other, forming an "X." I assumed I had determined the edge of her field and marked the spot by placing a pencil on the floor where I stood.

I approached her a second time without the rods, this time with my eyes closed, my hands in front of me, palms out, to see if I could feel the edge of her field. When it felt like I had encountered a large balloon, I stopped. Opening my eyes, I glanced down at the floor... and there at my feet was the pencil! I was astonished at this sudden awareness of a previously unknown part of the body.

I continued my energy-field experiment by asking my friend to imagine a happy event in her life. Again, I approached her with the rods, and this time they crossed about six feet from her body, providing confirmation that her field had doubled in size. My friend had kept her eyes closed as I moved toward her, and indicated she could actually sense when I encountered her field, which coincided with the crossing of the rods.

At the time, I was just at the beginning of discovering for myself, as a Western-trained healthcare professional, what other cultures have always known. I would soon learn about other energy systems and structures of the human body, including the chakras.

The Chakras

The word "chakra" is an ancient Sanskrit word meaning "wheel of light." References to these energy centers exist in cultures throughout the world. In modern practices, the most commonly recognized system includes seven major chakras that are paired with the seven layers of the human energy field. These cone-shaped vortices of spinning energy emanate from seven points along the central axis, and are connected through energy channels called nadis, a Sanskrit word meaning "movement."

While the central nadi lies within the spinal cord, two other main nadis surround and intersect with the chakras, crossing the central axis four times. The anatomical arrangement of the three main nadis is depicted in the caduceus, the symbol used to represent the American Western medical profession—two serpents criss-crossed around a central staff. From the central axis, each chakra projects outward, the large end of the cone opening out through the body from the pelvic floor to the crown of the head.

We gather information from the universal energy field through the chakras. Information-encoded waves of energy enter and leave the human system through each chakra, which act as our power centers for sensing energy and gaining an understanding of our environment. Through the chakras we communicate using the language of energy. Beginning with the energy center located at the pelvic floor and ascending to the crown of our head, the seven major chakras are our energy centers for sending and receiving information about our life force, creativity, personal power, love, expression, intuition, and spiritual connection, in that order.

The wavelengths of the vibrational frequencies of the seven major energy centers correspond to the seven colors in the visible spectrum seen in a rainbow, and to the seven musical notes of the C scale. Starting with the first chakra and ending with the seventh, the wavelengths of each energy center correlate with the colors red, orange, yellow, green, blue, indigo, and violet, and with the musical notes C, D, E, F, G, A, and B. The colors and sounds of the wavelengths of our chakras can be seen and heard by those having high coherence with the universal energy field.

An aspect of the flow of energy through the nadis and chakra system is the energy of consciousness, known as *kundalini*, a Sanskrit word meaning "sleeping snake." In the East, kundalini energy is thought to lie dormant at the base of the spine, like a slumbering serpent, until it rises through the central nadi and activates each chakra in ascending order. Enlightenment is said to occur when all seven energy centers become fully activated.

In the East, the energy centers are thought to develop and open chronologically during our lifetime. The first chakra is said to develop between the age of 1 and 8, the second chakra from age 8 to 14, the third chakra from age 14 to 21, the fourth chakra from age 21 to 28, and the fifth chakra from age 28 to 35. There is no association between age and development of the sixth and seventh energy centers.

Our state of health and well-being is reflected in the functioning of our energy centers. The more open the chakra, the more unobstructed the energy flow and the healthier we are. In the next chapter, we will look at the function of the chakras, the nadis, and kundalini energy in more detail as they relate to blockages in these energy systems.

Besides the major chakras, there are also numerous minor chakras, primarily in our joints. These secondary energy centers can also be found in the palms of the hands, from which energy flows with the intention of healing, and the nipples, which in women open during early pregnancy and from which energy flows to an infant during breastfeeding.

The existence of these energy centers has been documented

by scientists, most notably UCLA professor and research scientist Dr. Valerie Hunt, who has been studying and verifying the chakras for over twenty years. Dr. Hunt has recorded radiation emanating from locations in the body associated with the chakras. By measuring and analyzing the frequencies of this electromagnetic radiation emitted from the body and from each chakra, Dr. Hunt has been able to scientifically validate observations made by healing practitioner Rosalyn Bruyere of the chakras and the related layers of the field, including the colors that correspond to each wave frequency.

By the time I began learning about energy centers, I had at least let go of enough resistance to be curious. Like my dowsing rod experiments with the human energy field, I conducted my own investigations in detecting the chakras, first with a dowsing tool called a pendulum, then with my hands, and later with my developing inner sight and hearing. Various objects can be used as a pendulum, including a crystal, pendant, or ring hanging from a length of chain. I prefer a wooden pendulum shaped like an acorn, suspended from about six inches of string.

By holding the end of the string and allowing the pendulum to hang over the area associated with a chakra, and observing the movement of the pendulum, information can be obtained regarding the state of the chakra. Depending on the pattern of the pendulum's movement, whether clockwise, counterclockwise, vertical or horizontal, one can determine whether the energy of the chakra is blocked or flowing. The speed at which the pendulum moves, and the size of the spin, indicates whether the chakra is weak or energized. Barbara Brennan, physicist and healing practitioner, details this process of energy center "diagnosis" with the use of a pendulum in her book *Hands of Light: A Guide to Healing Through the Human Energy Field*.

Information I gathered about the energy field and the chakras through dowsing tools was soon augmented in a very personal way. During the time that I was experiencing infertility, I had a spontaneous vision while folding laundry, shortly after I had ovulated. I had been experiencing these instances of intuition while doing mundane chores since I was a teenager. The performing of menial tasks seemed to help me enter a mindful, meditative state. At first these experiences involved gut feelings and "knowings," but as I studied energy medicine, they expanded to inner visions and auditory messages. In this occurrence, an egg-shaped sphere of light appeared in my mind's eye, within a void of darkness. The exquisite color of the sphere was almost beyond description, a silvery-blue glow I had never seen in ordinary reality, as it only existed as intuitive information accessed from the universal energy field.

At the center of the sphere was an axis, and along that axis dots began to form, one at a time, until there were seven. Golden threads of light arched to connect from the top of the axis to the bottom in the same pattern seen when iron fillings on a piece of paper are held over a magnet. At first I didn't understand what this image was, or the significance. And then in an instant I knew—I was seeing the beginning of life forming within me, the energy systems of a developing embryo. The sphere and the golden threads were the electromagnetic energy field, and the dots were the beginning of the seven chakras forming along the core axis, a breathtaking sight.

Although I didn't know it at the time, the information I received in that intuitive moment was scientifically accurate. Dr. Harold Burr, Professor of Anatomy at Yale University School of Medicine, discovered an electrical axis in the human egg that becomes a guide for embryonic and fetal development after fertilization. Researchers have determined that energy patterns become established *before*, and are integral to the creation *of* the physical organs and tissues of the body. Physical development in the human embryo begins at the midline of the body and progresses in relation to this central axis. In this way, we see that *energy systems determine the very formation of our being.* And as we will learn in the next chapter, when this energy is blocked or wounded, *the result is illness.*

Unfortunately, the pregnancy I had seen in the vision abruptly ended only weeks later, as did many others. I was left heartbroken and angry that I was shown images of the beginning of life, only for that life to seemingly be taken away. It would take time to comprehend the gift I had been given, time marked by cycles of loss and grief. Working with that grief would become a powerful catalyst for growth and learning. How our wounds can become a vehicle for personal transformation will be explored further in later chapters, but for now, let's continue our survey of the human energy systems.

The Meridians

The earliest known references to meridian therapies date back over 5,000 years, originating in China. Since that time, knowledge of Traditional Chinese Medicine (TCM) has gradually spread around the globe, arriving last in the West. TCM is a complex health system that includes the meridians and the hundreds of acupuncture points that lie on them, as well as treatment principles based on the five elements believed to make up the world, the cycles of nature and life, the oppositional forces of yin and yang, and the internal and external causes of disease.

The twelve standard meridians are actually a single pathway

that transports energy throughout the body. Each meridian is a segment of this pathway as it appears near the surface of the body in the connective tissues. These segments are accessed through acupoints.

In addition to the twelve standard meridians, there are several secondary meridian group, including a deeper system of eight meridians referred to as "vessels." In contemporary treatment systems, two of these vessels, the Governor vessel and the Conception vessel, are included with the twelve main meridians. Together, these pathways function like the body's electrical system.

A number of scientific studies have documented the meridian system, using heat-sensing thermography, electronics, and through the work of French researcher Dr. Pierre de Vernejoul, radioactives. Using gamma-camera imaging, de Vernejoul and his research team injected radioactive isotope into acupoints and other random sites in the skin. Only the tracer injected into acupoints moved, and it did so precisely along meridian pathways. In healthy individuals, the isotope moved faster than research subjects who were ill. This confirms a principle of TCM, that disturbance in the energy flow through meridians impacts health and can lead to illness and disease.

There are many ways to work with these energy channels, from acupuncture, the placement of needles directly into acupoints, to acupressure, the use of manual pressure directly on acupoints, to more modern techniques involving finger tapping of acupoints.

Donna Eden, a therapist who works in energy medicine, explores the human energy field, the chakras, the meridians, and other lesser known energy systems in *Energy Medicine: Balancing Your Body's Energies for Optimal Health, Joy, and Vitality*. In her work with thousands of individuals, Eden has developed numerous self-help techniques for working with the meridians, including tracing the meridians with the fingers, as well as holding, massaging, and tapping on acupoints.

In 1980, Roger Callahan, Ph.D., clinical psychologist, discovered that finger tapping on an acupoint at the end of a meridian rapidly alleviated a long-standing phobia in a client who had not responded to traditional psychotherapy. Based on this finding, coupled with his study of quantum theory and Eastern principles, he developed "Thought Field Therapy," or TFT.

Callahan formulated numerous tapping formulas, which he called "algorithms"—individual protocols for tapping specific acupoints located on the ends of meridians. Each algorithm contained a fixed sequence of tapping, incorporated with eye movements from the field of neurolinguistic programming (NLP) to enhance effectiveness. His healing algorithms for the low vibrational states of trauma, anger, guilt, anxiety, panic, rage, addictive urges, phobias, depression, obsession, guilt, shame, embarrassment, jet lag and physical pain can be found in *Tapping the Healer Within: Using Thought Field Therapy to Instantly Conquer Your Fears, Anxieties, and Emotional Distress.*

Building upon Callahan's discoveries, Gary Craig, Stanford engineer and Certified Master NLP practitioner, determined that the effectiveness of TFT was not dependent on the order in which the acupoints were tapped. Based on this discovery, he founded "Emotional Freedom Techniques," or EFT, by combining all of Callahan's algorithms into a single generic tapping protocol. Rather than using a different algorithm for each issue or "negative" emotion, the "basic recipe" of EFT can be used for virtually any emotional or physical issue, as detailed in the handbook *The*

EFT Manual. Craig's finding that the sequence of tapping is irrelevant has been borne out by the millions who have received relief through EFT, and makes sense given the interconnected nature of the meridians and other energy systems of the body. The meridians, as they appear in the head, upper body, and hand, are depicted in an acutapping chart that can be found in the appendix.

To further our understanding of how energy systems determine the formation of our physical bodies, let's explore how the seen and unseen parts of the body are actually one.

Interdependent Systems

As we learned in chapter 2, the physical body systems work together as one harmonious whole. The immune system, nervous system, endocrine system, circulatory system, and all other systems of the physical body work together in concert, coordinated through waves of energy. In the same way, the energy field, chakras, meridians, and other energy structures are interdependent and in constant communication through the flow of energy through these systems. In turn, all the systems of the body work together, both the physical and energetic, in a cohesive, integrated fashion. As all of life is fundamentally energetic, in effect, *all* body systems are energy systems.

We have learned that the development of the subtle and physical body begins at the midline of the body—the *core*. To deepen our understanding of the significance of the body core, I would like to present information to you regarding the *craniosacral system*. This system inhabits the midline of the body—the central axis where the development of the body first begins, and around which the body and its energy systems organize. From my experience and perspective, it is in this core of the body where our physical, emotional, mental, and spiritual selves converge. In *Craniosacral Therapy and the Energetic Body: An Overview of Craniosacral Biodynamics*, Roger Gilchrist refers to this core of the body as "the center of the psyche, the dwelling place of the spirit."

All energy systems emanate from this core of the body. The governor and conception vessel meridians of Traditional Chinese Medicine, the central nadi that connects the chakras of the Hindu healing system, and the structures of the craniosacral system all inhabit the midline of the body. The spinal fluid of the craniosacral system flows through the same space as the central nadi. When I am working with a client, the energy flow through the central nadi and the flow of spinal fluid through the dural tube are perceived as *one*.

The craniosacral system encompasses the membranes, bones, nerves, and fluids at the core of a human being. Through the central axis between two poles, energy flows through these core structures of the craniosacral system: the dural membrane, cranium, spine, central nervous system, and cerebrospinal fluid. The dural membrane encases the brain and spinal cord, creating a container for the cerebrospinal fluid. Floating within the spinal fluid, the nerve roots of the central nervous system that control all body physiology are bathed by this vital fluid. The bones of the craniosacral system, the cranium and the spine, are attached to the dura and encompass the two poles of the body.

The cerebrospinal fluid circulates throughout the craniosacral system in a rhythmic pattern that William Sutherland, osteopathic doctor and researcher, referred to as *primary respiration*. Within the dural membrane, spinal fluid rises upward toward the brain, and then recedes toward the sacrum. This two-phased continuous cycle of movement is similar to the rising and falling of the chest in respiration. In his research and practice, Dr. Sutherland noted functional, emotional and cognitive difficulties when this natural motion was impeded.

The two phases of the spinal fluid movement are reflected in the subtle widening and elongating, followed by the narrowing and shortening of the craniosacral structures of the body. This subtle movement is most apparent when cradling the cranium and sacrum in the hands, but with practice can be palpated anywhere in the body.

This movement of spinal fluid follows the pattern of embryonic cell development. In the embryo, the nervous system is the first body system to form, created through cells that migrate toward the midline and then upward toward the head. Throughout the lifespan, the cells of the central nervous system pulsate in unison in this pattern set during initial development.

Dr. Sutherland was more interested in the *driving force* behind the rhythmic movement of the craniosacral system—a force he called *the Breath of Life*—more so that the movement itself or the structures of the system. In time, he came to appreciate how this energetic force is the essence of life, the same conclusion reached by quantum physicists.

Franklyn Sill founded an approach to craniosacral therapy called Craniosacral Biodynamics. His two-volume work, *Craniosacral Biodynamics,* provides a very thorough accounting of the profound implications for healing that can be accessed by working with this core system where the oneness of body, mind, and spirit is most evident.

In addition to Dr. Sutherland and Franklyn Sill, osteopath Dr. John Upledger has contributed much to the research of craniosacral dynamics and advancement of the field of craniosacral therapy. His biomechanical therapeutic approach to disturbances in the craniosacral system has led to greater public awareness and wider availability of craniosacral therapy.

As I began practicing therapy specifically for the craniosacral system, I learned firsthand the integrative nature of energy systems in my work with clients. Even if I used only craniosacral therapy in a session, the energy flow through previously blocked chakras would be restored, as if I had used a modality particularly for working with the energy centers. Likewise, when I began practicing acutapping, the interdependence of energy systems of the body became evident once again. Even if I used only acutapping in a session, tapping on the ends of meridians, I found that a restricted craniosacral rhythm would improve in ways I thought only craniosacral therapy could effect. However, while all energy systems are fundamentally interconnected, there is no single approach that will address all issues and one healing therapy does not replace another.

While I have found acutapping to be the most effective technique to address a phobia, such as the fear of public speaking, other modalities are also helpful. Similarly, when working with an individual who is suffering from, for example, a post-concussion headache, I have found craniosacral therapy to be the most effective approach, although again, any energy-based healing approach would be beneficial. It is for this reason that I prefer to practice and integrate a variety of modalities, using my intuition to determine which would work best for a client's issue, or for a specific aspect of that issue.

In the concussion example, I would use craniosacral therapy to alleviate the injury-related restrictions in the craniosacral system causing the headache. But to more completely address those issues, I would include acutapping in the same session for any emotional effects related to the accident that caused the injury. In addition, if a client is working with another practitioner in a modality I don't practice at the same time they are working with me, the effects are synergistic and especially helpful in severe and complex issues.

The important thing to know is this: Healing begins in the core. We will be expanding on this vital concept throughout this book.

Now that we know more about the anatomy of our energy systems, let's continue our journey of learning about energy medicine by exploring the forms that energy blockages within these systems can take and how they result in poor health and illness.

Even though knowledge of energy systems and how they impact health may not have been a part of my experience or education, this knowledge is my birthright, and as I read this book I am restoring that deficit.

Even though I may have been unaware of my own energy field or energy centers, I know that I am free to conduct my own personal research by exploring my subtle body, if I so choose.

ENERGETIC DISRUPTIONS

"...the cause of every negative emotion and
most physical symptoms is a block or disruption
in the flow of energy..."

—GARY CRAIG

OUR ESSENTIAL NATURE is to gravitate toward health. If we are moving in the direction of physical, emotional, mental, or spiritual "illness," a blockage in our energy systems is indicated.

In chapter 3, the concept of energy blockages was introduced through Steven's story. In his first session, blocked energy had revealed itself as the arrested energy pattern behind his eyes, which felt like an encapsulated "cyst" of compacted, frozen energy. But this was only a first "layer" of the energy disturbances that he carried. In later sessions, other blockages in other energy systems would reveal themselves.

In fact, these disturbances in energy can take many forms. I want to tell you about some of them here.

"Blockages" in our Energy Systems

In the last chapter, we looked at scientific studies that have documented how our energy is organized and the relationship between illness and disturbed energy flow. These disruptions can vary from complete arrest to decreased flow, and can include damage of the energy structures themselves.

I must tell you: The field of energy medicine is still in its infancy and the terminology to explain "pathologies" in the energy field is just emerging. I and other healing practitioners use descriptive terms to convey what we experience when we work with clients. Blockages in our energy systems cannot be described in the same way that, say, a conventional medical doctor might describe an illness in the body. This is because western-trained doctors view the body and its systems in their component parts, whereas the energy medicine practitioner sees the human as a whole, with all the energy systems interrelating and flowing into and out of one another. Our bodies are a continuous energy system, and therefore cannot be reduced to a localized malfunction. Describing energy blockages as isolated entities is like trying to relate the nature of the ocean by describing one wave.

Relating examples for each type of blockage creates the same difficulty as relating the blockages themselves, because in reality a single energy disturbance cannot be isolated from the whole of a client's issue. Blockages in the functioning of our energy systems always appear as a constellation of disturbances related to inter-dependent factors that can be complex. In the same way, it is possible to depict the spherical Earth in a flat map of the world, but that map is not entirely accurate.

Information about the state of a client's energy comes through *as a whole*, with emphasis on how I can best work with them at that particular moment. The focus of the healing session lies in being a healing *presence*, while letting the client's response guide me—rather than cataloguing each individual disturbance. This is why I generally don't do "aura readings" or "chakra readings," because when the focus is on listing specific blockages, it can actually detract from the healing process.

However, in order to convey information about energy blockages through the medium of this book, I will take information out of context, breaking it down energy system by energy system. My intention is that by the time you finish reading this book the whole picture will emerge for you.

Those are the caveats. Nonetheless, in order to convey these "energy pathologies" in a sensible, linear fashion, I will categorize them by energy system, using the most commonly accepted energy systems discussed in chapter 4. Each energy disturbance will be illustrated by characters I will introduce in this chapter. We will be revisiting some of these characters in later chapters as we explore other energetic concepts.

As we discuss these energy blockages, please keep in mind that the formation of these blockages happens unconsciously. If you recognize yourself in any of the characters, know that you have done nothing "wrong." By the same token, also know that although the creation of these energetic disturbances is an unconscious process, we are not helpless to change them. Everyone has the power to make healing choices, but doing so requires awareness—awareness that begins with an understanding of energy blockages.

Auric Blocks

In *Hands of Light,* healing practitioner Barbara Brennan details the forms energy disturbances can take in the human energy field, also known as the aura, such as holes, tears, rips, leaks, and lesions. Energy disturbances also appear as areas of stagnant or blocked energy, depleted or low energy, areas of excessive accumulation of energy, and changes in the shape of the field.

I obtain information about the state of a client's field by accessing the universal energy field while in a meditative state. This information contains visual and auditory information, which I augment through my kinesthetic senses, using my hands to feel the shape of the field, and looking for any unusual energy movement.

Those who have natural coherence with the universal energy field, or who have developed such coherence through practice, can perceive these disruptions in energy. But for those who are unable to perceive these disturbances, how do we know they exist? Because it is reflected in how we *feel.* The words we use to describe how we feel provide a clue to the state of our energy systems. In addition, these energy disturbances have been documented using Kirlian photography and aura imaging technology.

As I studied energy medicine, I began to become aware of these cysts, tears, holes and other disturbances in energy systems. At first it was difficult for me to trust my intuitive senses, as these occurrences were so far outside my accepted view of reality. Corroborating client symptoms with these disturbances provided some confirmation of the existence of energy blockages. In addition, aura imaging technology now provides a more practical way of documenting energy disruptions.

Guy Coggins, a Kirlian photography researcher, sought to improve upon aura photography in the 1970s, inventing a series of cameras, the most recent of which is the Aura Camera 6000, which takes color Polaroid pictures, and the WinAura computerized system, which displays videos on a computer monitor while the subject is in motion. Coggins used knowledge of the human energy field from ancient cultures, energy medicine practitioners, and scientific research in his aura imaging technology. This aura imaging system is highly sensitive and capable of detecting even minute changes in the subtle body.

No camera exists that can take a photo of the actual energy field around a living being. Rather, the images recorded with aura imaging technology are created in a similar way to our own human imaging system. Just as the lens of the eye converts wave information into images, aura imaging systems convert biofeedback data received from a hand sensor into colorful images. These systems have been calibrated using input from sensitives who are able to see the bands and colors of the human energy field. Aura camera operators around the world are beginning to record energy field disturbances in photographs and videos.

I want to give you word-pictures of the auric disturbances I have encountered, and then let the clients describe how these disturbances were created. It is amazing how they correlate.

Rips or Tears. When an individual has surgery, gives birth, or sustains a physical injury, it is not just the physical body that is cut or injured. The subtle body is equally affected, resulting in rips or tears that can extend through the layers of the field and can persist long after the physical body has healed. When I encounter a tear that has compromised the integrity of the field, it feels like I am passing my hand over a puncture in an inflated object and air is seeping out—although this is energy escaping, not air, so the tactile feeling is more subtle.

Two clients presented with similar disruptions in the integrity of their energy fields, tears from different causes. A year after giving birth to her second daughter, Whitney was still mentally and physically exhausted. Her field had a scattered appearance with a diffuse, uncontained feel to it. Indeed, she described herself as feeling scattered and depleted, even when the baby was sleeping through the night. Another client, Sophie, was experiencing extreme fatigue after weight loss surgery. I noted the deflated appearance of her field before she even described herself as feeling "deflated."

Not everyone who gives birth or has surgery will have these difficulties. In both of these cases, there were extenuating circumstances. The premature birth of Whitney's daughter was traumatic, due to her daughter's long stay in intensive care. Sophie had complications related to severe nutritional deficiencies that resulted from her gastric bypass surgery.

Misshapen. Even if an injury or impact does not sustain a tear in the field, it can disturb the shape and orientation of the field. When I first worked with Brooke, her energy field appeared shifted to the left and was no longer oriented to the central axis. She complained of feeling off-balance, dizzy, and "beside herself" ever since an auto accident in which her car—and her energy field—were struck from the right. In the nine years since the accident, she had gone from one physician to another seeking treatment for her illness symptoms, but had received no relief.

Holes, leaks. It's not just physical injury or surgery that can create these holes, leaks, and distortions in the field. Nonphysical emotional, mental and spiritual trauma can create them as well. Nora's field was leaking, collapsed, and unable to contain energy. She had felt "flat" for years after receiving the traumatic news that her brother had died in a car accident. Jim had a hole in his field over his abdominal area. His volatile relationship with his father had recently come to a head in a heated argument fueled by alcohol. Jim's father blamed him for his mother's abandonment of the family when Jim was a young teen. "My father's words cut like a knife. I literally felt eviscerated," said Jim.

Stagnant, dull. Medications, food, and lack of sleep also impact energy flow in our fields. Audrey's field appeared "dull," with areas of stagnant energy that I perceived as gray in color. She was taking medications to cope with the emotional aftermath of her second pregnancy loss. Although the medications had suppressed the depression and anxiety, Audrey felt sluggish and dull.

Sophie had dark and cloudy areas in her field that were almost nauseating to my senses. She was consuming artificially sweetened and highly processed diet food products that her physician had recommended after gastric bypass surgery. Sophie described feeling sluggish and "toxic," with a foul taste in her mouth, as if she had been poisoned. I noticed the vibrancy of her field and the flow of energy through her energy systems was significantly diminished from previous sessions.

Flares. Physical, emotional, mental and spiritual issues can always be seen in our energy fields. During Deidra's healing session, flashes of red energy appeared over areas she indicated were painful. Deidra had been diagnosed with both chronic fatigue syndrome and fibromyalgia, and described her pain as "flaring up" in various places throughout her body.

Foggy, depleted. Deidra's field was contracted and close to her body, and had a foggy appearance. She described her life with chronic fatigue syndrome as "limited," feeling "small," pulled in, energy-depleted, and mentally foggy.

Lesions. Usually individuals seek my help after they have developed a significant physical, emotional, mental, or spiritual issue, but sometimes I see a disturbance in the energy field *before* it has caused a significant issue. One lady came to me curious about energy work, with general issues of stress and anxiety. I became concerned for her when I saw an area of black in her field over her right breast, with black tentacle-like projections reaching into the breast. When I suggested she scan her body for tension or any unusual sensation, she admitted that she had been feeling a strange aching and pulling sensation in her right breast for months that caused her anxiety. Although all the medical tests her physician ordered had come back negative, she remained concerned. After working with deeper emotional issues that surfaced during the session, and techniques that worked directly with the energy blockages, I referred her to a vibrational remedies practitioner. It's impossible to know if she would have developed a disease in the breast, such as cancer, had she not received energy medicine, but it is known that disturbances in energy precede the development of disease and illness.

Blocked, compacted. Barbara Brennan has developed a system of classifying energetic blockages in the field based on their causes. Brennan describes suppression and compaction blockages that result from pushing down feelings, and blockages that function like armor to avoid and immobilize feelings. Katie, who we met in chapter 2, had these kinds of blockages. She carried excess weight in the abdominal area and her energy was very compacted.

Distortion. Our body shape does provide us with information as to the status of our energy systems. While we may assume that body shape changes are an inevitable result of aging, changes we see in our bodies over time are a reflection of the predominant state of our energy. Individuals whose energy field is top-heavy tend to carry weight in the upper part of the body and have thin legs. A person who is grounded but may be having difficulty maintaining a spiritual connection can have a field that is smaller at the top and bigger at the bottom, with a thin upper body and arms and thick legs and hips. Those who are chronically ill with a small, collapsed field can have small, frail bodies.

Prickly, withdrawn, shifted. Barbara Brennan's energy block categories include blockages that result in energy leaks that cut off flow of energy into the limbs, and disturbances that result from a defensive reaction. Blockages that form from feeling attacked or unsafe distort the natural egg-shape of the field, resulting in a field that can become sharp and prickly, withdrawn and pulled upward, or shifted to the left or right. I have seen these types of blockages in Deidra, the lady with chronic fatigue and fibromyalgia I referred to earlier in this chapter. Deidra had been sexually abused as a child, and her arms felt chronically tense, heavy and weak. Her father had attacked her at night in her sleep while holding down her arms. As an adult, Deidra's field was pulled upward and she had no energy flowing into her arms.

Many of these auric disturbances have been documented through aura imaging technology. In photos and videos taken with these systems, camera operators have recorded flares, gaps associated with holes and tears, and dark areas, as well as the changes that occur during an energy medicine therapy session. These images depict the transfer of energy between practitioner and client, even when the two are separated by distance. Aura imaging systems have also recorded the response of the client's field during a healing interaction, from contracted and dull, to expanded and vibrant. In "chakra mode," the WinAura system has recorded disturbances in the chakras as well.

Chakral Blocks

The first chakra of Jocelyn, who we met in chapter 1, was not spinning. This energy center is situated at the base of the spine, opens out through the pelvic floor and is related to life force. The reasons why became clear as she described her difficulty with lack of passion for anything in her life, including a lack of sexual desire. She felt numb, ungrounded, "all in her head," and stuck in the past. This energy center is also called the "base" or "root" chakra, as it is connected to the legs, which serve as our "roots." From this base, energy flows upward toward the crown of the head.

As a side note, I want to mention that issues with the first chakra seem rampant here in the West. This is a reflection of cultural leanings and issues. Healing practitioner Rosalyn Bruyere, for one, has noted the energy fields of Americans include a wide range of issues stemming from blockages in the first chakra.

First chakra. If you imagine the chakra system as a flowering plant, with the roots representing the first chakra, the flower representing the seventh or crown chakra, and the pairs of leaves as the remaining chakras connected to the stem, or central nadi, you can see how a problem in the root of the plant would impact all the other structures of the plant. Given this cultural pattern of issues in the root energy center, we can see how the high rates of cancer, arthritis, colitis, Alzheimer's disease, inflammatory disease, heart disease, high blood pressure, and sexual dysfunction seen in the West *all* relate to blocks in the first chakra caused by suppression. We'll discuss the effects of suppression at greater length in chapter 8. (see figure 5-1)

This cultural phenomenon of first chakra issues includes the gynecological issues that so many Western women have—infertility, endometriosis, menstrual irregularities, difficulties in menopause, and high rates of Cesarean Section and forceps-assisted births. Personally, I have also noted energy blockages in the first chakra in women who have been diagnosed with fibromyalgia and chronic fatigue syndrome.

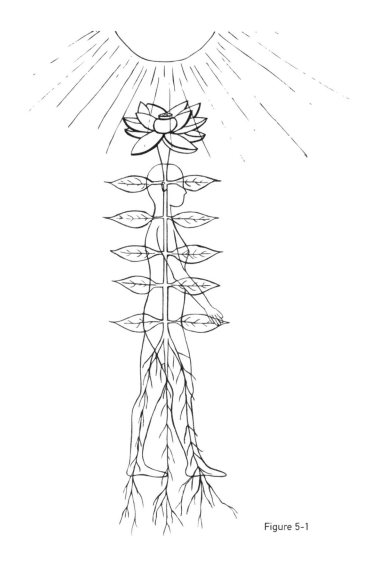

Figure 5-1

The most significant aspect of this blocked root energy center phenomenon in the West is the impact on kundalini energy. If we look at the stories presented in the first three chapters of this book—involving Jocelyn and myself, Katie, and then Steven— each one of these stories was an illustration of living in a state of dormant kundalini energy. For each individual, the lack of body awareness, the emotional numbness, the feeling of being "half-dead," the engaging in compulsive activity in an attempt to feel more alive—all were a function of dormant kundalini.

To understand how a blocked first chakra creates dormant kundalini, we have only to look at the flowering plant analogy. When the root energy center is blocked, this would be like a plant with a blockage at the base of its stem, disconnecting the roots from the rest of the plant. When the first chakra is blocked, kundalini energy is unable to rise through our "stem," or central nadi, to the "leaves," the remaining energy centers, or open the "flower" or crown chakra.

Energy center imbalances can take various forms. Chakras can be clogged or disfigured, and have frequencies that are weak and undercharged, or jarring and overcharged, as well as being out of synchrony with the rest of the energy system. Energy centers can also become overdeveloped or underdeveloped when we overuse or underuse one way of relating to the world, as we shall see when we examine chakral blockages in greater detail.

To be in a fully balanced state with all chakras activated is to be in a kundalini-awakened state. This process of enlightenment that occurs when kundalini energy rises and fully activates all the energy centers can happen spontaneously, through personal spiritual practices, or in the course of healing work. However, forcing kundalini to rise through intensive meditation practices before one is ready can create a full-blown experience that overloads the nervous system and can cause a break with reality.

The concept of kundalini awakening can be difficult for Westerners to comprehend, as the kundalini experience was rarely seen outside of the East until the 1970s, when our culture began to focus on consciousness. It is still an uncommon experience for a Westerner. We've already explored the events behind this wide-spread Western kundalini dormancy that began with the influence of Descartes philosophy, Newtonian physics, and culminating in the publication of the Flexner Report. Other implications of the resulting split between science and spirituality, self and nature, and the body into parts will be discussed in later chapters, in particular how it has contributed to a pattern of separatism and suppression in our Western culture that is a major factor in the formation of blockages in our energy systems. But for now, let's continue our exploration of energy center blockages with examples of blocks in each chakra.

Due to the interconnected nature of energy systems, it is unlikely that only one energy center would become blocked. However, in order to illustrate these blockages, in the following story examples, I will focus on only one chakra at a time.

Second chakra. The energy of the second chakra is womb-like. In the process of healing this energy center, we can have pregnancy dreams that represent the gestating of new ideas and expressions of our creativity. Likewise, an actual pregnancy can be a time of intense growth for both mother and father, with self gestated along with the baby.

As I worked with Audrey, the lady experiencing depression and anxiety after a pregnancy loss, I had a vision of a small version of her curled up in her own womb, a metaphor for healing through gestating ourselves. Her second chakra, the energy center related to creativity located between the pubic bone and the navel, was blocked. Audrey described feeling like her creativity had "dried up," and as if the "sweetness" had gone out of her life after her second miscarriage, a tragedy that had deeply affected her state of being and her creative work as an interior designer. In addition, her lower back was chronically tight and she felt emotionally deadened.

Third chakra. Jim's third energy center, the chakra related to personal power which is located in the region of the solar plexus, was not spinning and looked smashed flat. When his wife admitted her extramarital affair, he had felt as if he were "punched in the gut," and had been plagued with nausea and frequent stomach aches ever since. He felt helpless and powerless after receiving this devastating news and his sense of self was rocked. "I don't even know who I am anymore," said Jim.

Fourth chakra. Instead of being cone-shaped, Vanessa's fourth energy center, the heart chakra located in the center of the chest, was underdeveloped and shriveled. It resembled a flower that had collapsed and closed its petals, drooping on its stem. Vanessa was raised by parents who had little time for her. She never felt loved or cared for as they were unaffectionate and uninvolved in her life. As an adult, Vanessa had difficulty taking in love and affection and her chest felt sore and "bruised" at times when she didn't feel loved.

Fifth chakra. Claire's fifth chakra, located in the center of the throat and governing communication and expression, appeared pulled inside her physical body, rather than projecting out. As a child, Claire felt dominated by parents who constantly criticized her. As an adult, she was afraid of expressing herself to the people in her life for fear that they would reject her. Her throat frequently felt tight, and she was prone to sore throats and bouts of laryngitis that would cause her to literally lose her voice.

As noted earlier, the energy fields of Westerners tend to be "top-heavy." I have observed this phenomenon in my practice, and it has also been documented by healing practitioners such as Rosalyn Bruyere and Donna Eden. This distortion of auras in the West is related to our cultural tendency to relate to the world primarily on the mental level. This imbalance happens when we to try to "think" ourselves through issues, rather than connecting to our feelings. Our intellectual selves are overdeveloped, our emotional and spiritual selves underdeveloped, and we tend to be disconnected from our physical bodies. This "over-thinking" can clog and block the sixth and seventh chakras. We can change our thoughts, but it is vital to also work with our feelings, as doing so engages the lower energy centers.

Equally problematic is when the sixth and seventh chakras are the only energy centers that are open. I once worked with a fascinating woman who enjoyed sharing her mystical experiences, but her life was in complete disarray. Although she was highly aware spiritually, she had difficulty with basic activities of daily living, such as paying her bills, eating regular meals, and taking care of her health. All her lower energy centers were blocked.

Sixth chakra. The sixth chakra, also known as the "third eye," is located just above the bridge of the nose. This energy center is related to transcending our sense of self and receiving intuitive information. In individuals who are distrustful or frightened of their intuition the sixth chakra will appear blocked with energetic debris.

A child I worked with had been seeing things that frightened her for as long as she could remember. She called them spirits, and their appearance in her bedroom at night was especially distressing to her. I hadn't seen the young girl for a few months when her mother brought her in for an appointment when she was about ten years old. As I worked with the child, I noticed a pressure sensation in my own sixth chakra—often I do sense blocks in my clients through sensations in my own energy systems. I could see that the girl's sixth chakra was well-developed, but it looked like it had been capped off, like the cover of a camera lens. When I asked the girl if she still saw things that frightened her, she said no. She was not aware that she had stopped herself from seeing things. All she knew was that she no longer had those experiences.

In the West, many individuals block this chakra in childhood when they realize intuitive experiences aren't fully accepted in our society. We are born with the ability to perceive energy systems with our inner sight to varying capacities, but in the West few retain this ability into adulthood. While some do have childhood memories of seeing energy fields, for many it becomes blocked at such a young age that no memory of intuitive experiences remains.

Sometimes childhood memories of exploring energy surface during a healing session. For those who do remember, such memories may be attributed to a child's fanciful imagination, although imagination actually comes from our intuition.

Mandy verbally described and drew pictures of energy systems as a toddler. Although her mother supported and encouraged her experiences, cultural influences were stronger. As she grew and realized that others weren't aware of energy fields, she eventually suppressed her intuition and denied it ever existed. Even as a young adult, Mandy questions the validity of her early experiences, and out of a desire to "just be normal" and accepted by others, her sixth chakra was blocked, which effectively blocked the seventh, her connection to the spiritual realm.

Seventh chakra. In the religion Rita was raised in, she was expected to be subservient to men and suppress any aspects of herself that did not conform to church doctrine. Eventually she rejected God along with all organized religion, which left her feeling cut off and utterly alone. Although Rita desired spiritual awareness, the idea of "God" remained a mental concept and she was unable to experience the *feeling* of spiritual connection. Her seventh chakra, the energy center located at the crown of the head, was blocked.

Meridian Blocks

Disturbances in the meridians can take the form of excess flow of energy, referred to as *chi* in Traditional Chinese Medicine (TCM), diminished energy flow, and blockages. When a meridian is out of balance, the result is a constellation of physical, emotional, mental and spiritual symptoms that have been thoroughly catalogued in TCM.

The twelve main meridians are named for the bodily organs they serve, with the exception of the Triple Heater meridian, which is a three-branched pathway that governs the flow of energy through all the organs. The other eleven standard meridians are named after the gallbladder, liver, heart, small intestine, pericardium, stomach, spleen, lung, large intestine, kidney, and bladder.

As many meridians end at the fingertips, Kirlian photography can also be used to determine meridian imbalances. Fingertip photos have revealed a diminished or absent electrical coronal discharge at the location of an acupoint related to a specific meridian.

The goal of meridian therapies is restoring balance to the whole person within their environment. However, in the section that follows, examples of imbalances are isolated to a specific meridian. While all of the individuals in these examples had multiple issues and blockages in their energy systems, I have included only the issues that pertain to a particular meridian, and only the characteristics present for that individual. There are numerous other characteristics that one might see with a meridian imbalance, too many to include here. A more thorough description of all the qualities one might experience for each pathway imbalance can be found in *Bee in Balance: A Guide to Healing the Whole Person with Honeybees, Oriental Medicine, and Common Sense*, by acupuncturist and social worker Dr. Amber Rose.

Gallbladder meridian. Tess spoke in a soft voice, in contrast to the content of her speech, which was replete with descriptions of her anger and frustration. Her primary issues were arthritis and inflammation, and after she had an insight that unexpressed anger worsened her pain, she realized she needed to attend to deeper issues, not just medicate the pain. She spoke of feeling restless and having difficulty making decisions, and admitted that she was very judgmental of others. "I'm really a loving person, so I don't understand why I'm so critical of everyone." Her painful arthritis affected different joints at different times, but it was at its worst when she went to bed at night. Tess's pattern of issues pointed to an imbalance in the Gallbladder meridian. It was no coincidence that she had a history of gallstones and her gallbladder had been removed years earlier.

Liver meridian. Claire, the lady who felt constantly criticized as a child, cancelled several appointments in a row because of frequent infectious illnesses. "I keep getting sick," she lamented. "I just know my immune system isn't functioning properly." She also complained of feeling depressed and hopeless about her future, fatigue, and having trouble sleeping through the night, usually waking within a few hours of falling asleep. Claire's constellation of issues was consistent with an imbalance in the Liver pathway.

Heart meridian. In her initial session, Deidra described her life with chronic fatigue and chronic pain from fibromyalgia, and her history of childhood sexual abuse in a flat voice. "I just feel so empty, so overwhelmed with life," she added. Her history, voice, and words pointed to an imbalance in the Heart meridian.

Small Intestine meridian. Jocelyn had been in a series of relationships that were not good for her, and was confused about what to do. She also had digestive problems and complained of always feeling hot. Along with other blockages in her energy systems, Jocelyn had an imbalance in the Small Intestine pathway.

Heart Protector meridian. Vanessa, the lady who felt unloved by her parents, was afraid to share her opinions and dreams with her husband and friends out of fear of being hurt. As she lay on my healing table, I noticed that her hands and feet were very cold and pale. When I shared this observation with Vanessa, she reported that her circulation had always been poor, and that she persistently felt cold—all signs of an imbalance in the Pericardium, or Heart Protector meridian.

Triple Heater meridian. Helen had a lot of friends, but didn't feel close to any of them, which contributed to her sense of isolation while coping with infertility. When I laid my hand on her lower belly, just above her pubic bone, I noticed the sensation of coldness in her pelvis even though other parts of her body were hot. It was challenging to keep Helen comfortable during the session, as she alternated between feeling too warm, and then too cold. This pattern of issues made it clear that Helen's Triple Heater pathway was out of balance.

Stomach meridian. Whitney's third pregnancy was difficult with severe nausea, vomiting, and hypoglycemia. Despite the digestion problems, she was constantly hungry and craved sweets. "My husband and friends tell me I'm needy," she commented. Whitney's issues were indicative of an imbalanced Stomach meridian.

Spleen meridian. Deidra, who suffered from fibromyalgia and chronic fatigue, complained of feeling so tired and sluggish that she could barely walk across a room. Despite her limitations, any free time and energy she did have went toward the caretaking of others, not for herself. Deidra likely had an imbalance in her Spleen pathway.

Lung meridian. Jim had a troubled relationship with his father and had lung issues –suffering from asthma since he was a child, as well as bouts of bronchitis. He related that since he separated from his wife after her extramarital affair, he had lived alone and had few friends, but that he preferred it that way. His father, lung, and "loner" issues were consistent with a Lung meridian imbalance.

Large Intestine meridian. A gentleman I have worked with had spinal surgery years ago to repair damage from an accident at work. Unfortunately, his surgical outcome was poor, and he suffered from chronic pain, limited mobility, and compromised bowel function. His efforts to obtain a favorable settlement through the legal system had failed, which left him angry and bitter. In our work together, I noticed that while he was desperate to improve his situation, he was resistant to implementing changes that might actually do so, a quality that one might label stubbornness. Suggestions that he try an exercise for forgiveness, or implement a program of bowel care, were met with opposition. This combination of bowel issues and stubbornness, pervasive negativity, and an unforgiving attitude pointed to a Colon, or Large Intestine pathway blockage.

Kidney meridian. Another male client I have worked with who was born with abnormalities in his urinary system that required surgical intervention at a young age had chronic urinary tract infections throughout his life. I listened carefully as he described the anxieties and fears that he believed had kept him stuck and contributed to his lack of ambition and forward movement in his career. Taking into account his physical issues and fears, along with my observation of dark circles under his eyes and the premature graying of his hair, I knew that he had an imbalance in his Kidney meridian.

Bladder meridian. As I questioned this client further, I realized he also had an imbalance in the Bladder meridian. He described migraines that had been triggered by fear, a characteristic of an imbalance in both the Kidney and Bladder pathways. His chronic bladder infections, the slight swelling in his face, hands and feet, along with his propensity to overwork and push himself to the edge of his endurance, all indicated a blockage in the Bladder energy channel.

I want to point out that the characteristics I've described in each of these examples, such as neediness, stubbornness, and lack of ambition, are not criticisms. Although we may think of these characteristics as character flaws or negative personality traits, they are expressions of the blockages in our energy channels. Indeed, when people heal, they often describe feeling like a different person, as if they have gone through a personality change.

Although this survey of energy channel imbalances has been focused on specific meridians, for some techniques that work with the meridians, such as acutapping, determining which meridian is out of balance is not necessary to address the imbalance. By tapping on the ends of all of the meridians depicted in the illustration in the appendix, while staying focused on the distressing issue that the imbalance is creating, whichever meridian or meridians is the culprit will be addressed. This technique only takes minutes. Since the meridians are actually segments of the same continuous energy pathway, it is not even necessary to tap on the ends of all 12 meridians to achieve results.

In addition to blockages in the auric, chakral, and meridian energy systems, disruptions in energy can appear in the body core.

Core Blocks

Energy blockages in the subtle body are reflected in the function of the physical and energetic structures at the core of the body, the craniosacral system. These disruptions in energy can be palpated as disturbances in the symmetry, quality, amplitude and rate of the craniosacral rhythm.

Energy blockages can disrupt our natural orientation to midline, the core axis. In time, this misalignment can result in compensatory influences in our movement and function, and in limiting belief systems that arise from these physical limitations. These limitations include distortion of center of gravity, tight and shortened muscles, tendons, and ligaments, distortion of connective tissues, misaligned bones, restricted respiration, congestion of body fluids, and inflammation.

Orientation to one's core is the key to health. Being oriented to our core makes us feel whole and connects our core energetic processes. When we are oriented to a person, place, or thing outside of ourselves as our focus, this disruption in energy flow through the core is seen not just in our physical bodies, but in all areas of our life as we lose our spiritual connection and begin to rely on that "something else" to make us feel whole.

As a teenager, Mandy subconsciously thought her achievements would make her feel whole. But her outward-oriented focus
on grades, awards, and athletic feats left her feeling empty. Like
Dorothy in *The Wizard of Oz*, we always have the ability to "go
home," or to go within to connect with our essence. No matter
what traumas we have been through, we never lose the ability to
orient to the core of us and experience oneness with the universal
energy field—that spiritual connection in whatever way we define
it. As such, the feeling that we are separate is an illusion.

In the next chapter, we will explore other effects of trauma
on physical and energetic body systems and deeper aspects of core
blocks.

Regardless of the location of blockages in our energy systems,
the experience often feels like coming up against a wall.

Hitting the Wall

There is a broader aspect of energy blockages that seems to
be an almost universal experience—what we generally refer to as
"hitting the wall." When we use expressions like, "I feel like I'm
caught between a rock and a hard place," "I've painted myself
into a corner," "I feel hemmed in, blocked, stuck," or "I can't
move forward," we are speaking of the experience of encountering the "wall," the sensation of a blockage in our energy systems.

I want to make a point here: All these statements are coming
from intuition. Our bodies are trying to present us with information via the psyche. Most of us don't realize how deeply connected
we are to our intuition until we stop and listen to our own words.
Becoming aware of the mental images that depict bodily sensations as well as the body sensations themselves is the first step
toward healing the blocks in our energy systems.

In any case, the experience of the wall is associated with blockages in energy and is usually accompanied by a feeling of frustration. The area of our life where we feel frustrated gives a clue to the location of the blockage in our energy systems. But any blockage, regardless of location, can result in the experience of the wall.

Some of my clients have a mental image of an actual wall while thinking about areas of their life where they are unable to move forward, or during a healing session when we are working with an energy blockage.

When confronted with a wall, many people react with a desire to break through with their will, or to resist and fight the blockage. But there's always a reason the wall exists. Whether it is a result of past traumas, childhood experiences, or more current situations, "the wall" usually has been created out of fear and serves as protection. In the case of the later, the blockage may initially provide comfort, but in time it creates limitation and can become a source of frustration.

My personal experience of the wall took the form of a recurring vision of being trapped in a circular room where the wall wrapped around me, completely enclosing me. Before I began using energy medicine to treat my infertility, my frustration with the available conventional medical treatment options made me feel trapped. The circular room was like a prison in my mind, and its effects were felt throughout my life in my inability to move forward with anything. The circular room had doors that each represented family-building options, but none led me out of the room. I often wished I could smash my way out with a sledgehammer.

The door representing IVF (in vitro fertilization) was locked and I didn't have the "key," as IVF was neither covered by our health insurance nor within our financial means. The door representing my current Western medical treatment protocol was like a revolving door. Each month that I entered that door in the circular room of my mind, I would end up back in the room when the treatment failed, month after month, year after year. The door representing adoption could have completed our family, but I knew it wasn't going to heal the blocks. I felt I had to heal first before seriously considering that family-building option. After taking time off from conventional infertility treatment to heal the many disturbances in my energy systems, the blockages were released and a solution presented itself.

Healing the blockages in my energy was like being given the key that would lead me out of the circular room to greater health, and to my child. But what caused these blockages to form? As we shall see, disturbances in our energy systems are formed over a lifetime, and laid down in layers.

Even though recognizing myself in some of the examples of energy blockages in this chapter may have caused me to feel angst, I accept myself and feel gratitude for this emerging awareness.

Even though I now know that any blockages in my energy systems were unconsciously formed, now that I am conscious, I have the power to make healing choices to release these blockages. The knowledge to do so is being revealed to me moment to moment.

PART TWO:

DIS-EASE ESSENTIALS

The Evolution of Illness and Poor Health

*"The science of natural living and healing shows clearly
that what we call disease is primarily nature's effort to
eliminate morbid matter and to restore the normal
functions of the body; that the processes of disease
are just as orderly in their way as everything else
in nature; that we must not check or suppress them,
but co-operate with them."*

—HENRY LINDLAHR, MD

~ 6 ~

ENERGY WOUNDS

"...an attachment injury is an injury to the self,
an emotional or relational injury—a soul wound."

—TIM CLINTON, ED.D. AND GARY SIBCY, PH.D.

AS YOU MAY RECALL from the previous chapter, energy
blockages can appear in any or all of our energy systems and
negatively impact health. The question of how these blocks
are formed is the subject of this chapter. In order to explain
how these blockages in energy are formed, I would like to
deepen our discussion about them now.

These disruptions in energy are formed by interconnecting
factors that can be difficult to describe in a simple, logical way,
so I will begin with a likeness. If you wanted to obtain more
information on a topic through an Internet search, it is likely that
search would produce thousands of sources, and clicking on any
one of those search results could lead to a myriad of other sources

with these connections leading you in many different directions, including back to the original search sources—hence the name, "World Wide *Web.*" The factors involved in the formation of blockages in our energy systems are similarly interconnected, but for the sake of clarity, I will convey information about the evolution of energy disturbances as if the factors were sequential steps.

In my personal and professional work, I have found that energy blockages are formed by: *first,* a physically, emotionally, mentally, or spiritually injurious or traumatic experience; *second,* the shaping of beliefs based on the messages perceived from that experience; and *third,* judging and criticizing ourselves for the emotional response we have to a traumatic experience and suppressing that response.

For this reason, it's important to take a closer look at the traumas we all experience in life.

Now I admit that trauma can be an unpleasant subject to talk about. I often meet people who want to deny or avoid talking about anything negative or looking at "unpleasant stuff from the past." "What's the point? What good does that do?" they ask.

The truth is, in order to heal the blockages in our energy systems; we have to understand the role of trauma in their formation. Why? Because if we know the steps in the evolution of an energy blockage, we also know how to reverse the steps, release the block, and restore the natural flow of energy that is *vital to health.*

In later chapters, we will examine the steps to healing these energy blockages at their root, that is, the process of healing that was introduced in chapters 2 and 3 through Katie's and Steven's stories. But first, stay with me for an explanation of what constitutes trauma.

The Traumas of Life

We have seen how traumatic events such as surgery, a car accident, loss of a loved one, miscarriage, traumatic birth, violent argument, or discovery of an extramarital affair can create distur- bances in energy systems. The term "trauma" is usually associated with major events such as these. However, from my experience as an energy medicine therapist, the definition of trauma is much broader. Any physical, emotional, mental, or spiritual experience that is personally distressing, regardless of whether it is an isolated event or an ongoing state, can be traumatic *if it creates disruption* in our energy systems.

How do you know if an event or experience has caused a disruption in your energy systems?

Memories That Trigger Distress

If the memory of an event or a situation triggers a negative emotion or physical response, there is a disturbance in energy. No matter how trivial an event or situation may seem on the surface, no matter how irrational the emotional response may seem, and no matter how much time has passed since the event occurred—if certain situations trigger physical, emotional, spiritual, or mental distress, an energy disturbance is present in relation to that past trauma.

This distress can take the form of pain, discomfort, tension, tightness, anxiety, anger, fear, sadness, guilt, shame, negative thoughts, or a sense of disconnection.

Consider these examples and whether you can relate to one or more of them in some way.

Whenever Mandy receives a big bill in the mail, as soon as she opens it and sees the numbers, she feels "jolted." She becomes tense and anxious, and then tired and wiped out for the rest of the day. As a child, Mandy's family was plunged into poverty when her father's business went bankrupt and they lost everything. Mandy has a disturbance in her energy systems related to the trauma of losing her home and possessions.

When Whitney got on the hospital elevator to visit a friend, she was surprised to find herself in the sudden grip of anxiety. Her chest tightened, and she felt like she was going to cry. Years earlier, Whitney's second daughter had been born prematurely at that hospital and spent months in the intensive care nursery in critical condition. Whitney had a disruption in her energy systems related to the trauma of nearly losing her infant daughter years before.

Whenever Jim's estranged wife had expressed any unhappiness or dissatisfaction, Jim had experienced sudden guilt and anxiety, and felt compelled to fix whatever was causing the dissatisfaction. Jim carried a belief that everything was his fault and the expression of unhappiness and dissatisfaction in those around him made him feel unsafe. As a child, after his mother abandoned the family, he had to anticipate the needs of his alcoholic father and meet them in order to prevent violence and maintain safety. Jim had an energy disruption related to childhood trauma.

In some situations, the original trauma that caused the disturbance is unknown because the memory has either been consciously suppressed, or unconsciously suppressed, known as repression. Yet if symptoms are present, an energy blockage is indicated. Unexplained physical, mental, spiritual, or emotional symptoms can be related to trauma that may have occurred days, weeks, years, and even decades after a distressing experience. And although some therapies emphasize recapturing the memory of an event in order to heal it, this is not necessary in the process of energy healing.

It is likely anyone would be traumatized by a major dramatic event, but the degree to which they are traumatized rests largely on beliefs about ourselves and others, as well as the environment surrounding us in our early life.

The effects of these traumas on health, specifically those that occur in childhood, has been researched through the ongoing ACE Study (Adverse Childhood Experiences) conducted by the Center for Disease Control and Prevention and Kaiser Permanente. This study has found a strong correlation between childhood trauma and physical and behavioral health issues that are associated with the ten leading causes of death. Included in the ACE Study's list of nine household conditions that produce trauma—which a *majority* of adults have experienced at least one of—are childhood sexual trauma and the factors that produce insecure attachment, which I refer to as "attachment trauma." These distressingly common childhood traumas profoundly affect our beliefs, self-concepts, and health. In this chapter, we will begin our exploration of trauma by examining the affects of attachment trauma.

Please note that the labels I use for different types of trauma are for ease of explanation, and are not meant to be diagnostic or used as a means to define self. I know from personal and professional experience that once traumatized, we can easily identify with being a victim. I certainly don't want to add to that tendency by providing labels for victimization. Rather, I hope you see these categories as useful information meant to enhance awareness and understanding.

Attachment Trauma

The vast majority of clients I have worked with in the last fifteen years have suffered from attachment trauma during their childhood, including most of the client examples presented in this book. This injury results from being insecurely attached to a parental figure, particularly the mother, and is estimated to affect between 30 and 40 percent of adult Americans, a staggering number of individuals in an otherwise invisible epidemic. While those affected by attachment trauma may appear completely "normal" on the surface, they can suffer from pervasive unhappiness, anxiety, and anger.

How securely we attach to our parents has far-reaching effects throughout our lives, coloring relationships and self-image, determining emotional stability and confidence, and affecting our ability to feel compassion as well as how we react to stress and other traumas. Insecure attachment trauma occurs with inconsistent or rigid parenting, and not being in touch with an infant or child's needs. Attachment trauma can also be the result of separation from one or both parents as a result of illness, death, or other event.

Researchers have found that unpredictable parenting creates *ambivalent attachment*, characterized by resistant behavior in which the child eagerly desires contact with the parent, yet resists the parent's attempts to comfort. Rejecting parenting has been found to create *avoidant attachment*, characterized by indifference toward the parent. Both ambivalent and avoidant attachment involve suppressing emotions and suppressing the need for comfort. These suppressive responses are seen as a means to cope with the hurt and anger associated with inconsistency and rejection, as well as to protect self from further hurt. We will see how these two responses to attachment trauma—resistance and suppression—so prevalent in our society, are key factors in energy disturbances.

Lifelong Consequences

The Newtonian emphasis on separateness over connectedness that is engrained in the very fabric of Western society has deep influences on childcare practices. Despite compelling evidence produced from research conducted by British psychiatrist John Bowlby, and Canadian psychologist Mary Ainsworth, documenting that infants and children can experience rage, depression, and true mourning when separated from parents, the idea that one's well-being is dependent on being securely attached to a parent was strongly resisted in the West.

Western hospital policies that separate parents and children begin with birth. When I worked in a hospital obstetrics unit in the mid-1980s, mothers and babies staying together was still viewed as an unusual arrangement only available by special request. Although today most hospitals encourage mothers and infants to room together, newborns are still routinely separated from their mothers after birth for procedures and observation.

As late as the 1970s, it was hospital policy in the West to separate parents from hospitalized children for extended periods of time and to restrict the handling of babies and sick children out of the belief that doing so was dangerous and unhealthy, despite extensive documentation of the emotional damage these practices can cause.

Although hospitals no longer discourage visitation and handling of hospitalized infants and children, there are many adults living with the effects of unresolved childhood trauma from these policies. One such adult is Ted Kaczynski, also known as "The Unabomber." During the weeks that nine-month-old Ted was hospitalized for an allergic reaction, his parents were barred from holding him during the rare allowed visits. According to his mother, Ted became withdrawn and unresponsive to human contact after his hospitalization and was "never the same." Ted Kaczynski is currently serving a life sentence for the murders of three individuals carried out with bombs he created while living in self-imposed isolation.

Although Kaczynski's story is a rather extreme example of the effects of attachment trauma, it does give us an idea of the range of possible effects from separatist policies. While enforced parental abandonment can cause an individual to completely withdraw from human society and develop homicidal impulses, a less dramatic level of parental emotional neglect can create difficulty connecting with others and feeling empathy.

For decades American parents were warned by psychologists and pediatricians not to respond to their baby's crying in the belief that it would reinforce the behavior. In *Becoming Attached: First Relationships and How They Shape Our Capacity to Love*, clinical psychologist Robert Karen, Ph.D. writes, "It seemed contrary to nature and intuition, but behaviorist theory asserted that picking up the kid reinforced the crying, and if you did it enough you'd have a monstrous crybaby on your hands."

Behaviorist theory has been solidly disproven by the work of Mary Ainsworth. Through her research, we now know that crying is an infant attachment-seeking behavior, and trauma occurs when the cries of an infant go unheeded.

Parents were led to believe that negative behavior in a child, such as hatred and jealousy, had to be eliminated through punishment and shaming. This is especially true of parents of "baby boomers," children born during the post-World War II baby boom. Such strict upbringing has historically been considered the route to maturity in the West. However, just the opposite is true.

When the expression of natural conflicting love-hate feelings that all children have is blocked from expression, development becomes arrested. When shaming is used in parenting, the child can disown the parts of themselves that the parent disapproves of. This produces a state of kundalini dormancy and a lack of kundalini energy flowing through the central nadi that activates the chakras. Shaming also produces a state of low vibrational frequency incompatible with health.

It's important to understand an aspect of this disowning of parts of ourselves. Depth psychologists tell us that within each of us we have "parts." Everyone has aspects that they consider "dark," because we do not want to see ourselves in certain ways. For instance, we may not like to see ourselves as aggressive or causing conflict, and prefer to see ourselves as peacemakers. But then we may avoid conflict altogether by "allowing" another person to believe we agree with them while doing exactly what they would not like us to do—and we fail to see this passive-aggressive avoidance of that person for what it is, a hidden form of aggression.

Likewise, we prefer to see certain other traits in ourselves, so these traits are visible or in the "light." We may, for instance, feel compelled to be generous when we cannot afford to be, because it's important to keep seeing ourselves and have others see us as "generous." Both types of imbalances create huge amounts of energetic discord.

There are other aspects of this disowning of self. When we disown our "dark" parts, we keep these aspects of ourselves hidden. Psychologists call this hidden, disowned part the *shadow*, the part we reject, repress, and are ashamed of. When we repress parts of ourselves, we "project" these hidden parts on others, and then judge and criticize them for it, because it is safer to blame unacceptable behavior on others than to take responsibility for the unacceptable behavior in ourselves. Denying who we really are is considered a defense mechanism in psychology, a means of protection. Paradoxically, the shadow contains our greatest potential—a potential that becomes unleashed in the process of healing.

In later chapters we will further explore this *disowning*; the self-rejection that causes us to suppress parts of ourselves. Through stories of individuals who suppressed their true nature, we will see how doing so is detrimental to health.

Issues in Parenting

We have seen how being parented in a rejecting way can contribute to subsequently disowning aspects of ourselves. There are also other consequences to attachment trauma related to development.

The three stages of human development are dependence, independence, and then interdependence. At the beginning of life, we need to be completely dependent and merged with a parent figure. While this vital early experience of *oneness* is not required for one to become an independent adult, without it that adult is left with unmet dependency needs. These unmet dependency needs can prevent us from reaching full maturity and enlightenment—a state of *interdependence*, which is being dependent on others and independent *at the same time*. Ironically, in order to become an adult capable of healthy *detachment* from outcomes and ego, and free of projections, one needs to experience secure *attachment* in childhood.

In psychoanalysis, the "ego" is a mental construct for "self" as separate from others that begins in childhood based on what others reflect back to us. The formation of the ego is a necessary developmental step in differentiation. However, attachment to our ego selves effectively blocks us from our true selves. The process of healing core blocks includes *dropping* the ego self, also referred to as the "lower self," the "false self" or the "false center," in favor of our true being at our core—our authentic selves.

The goal of raising an independent, self-sufficient child is an important one, but it cannot be achieved by skipping the critical early experience of parental dependence. Infants need to experience complete dependence for approximately the first six months of their life. During the second half of the first year of their child's life, parents can begin to distinguish what their child *wants* from what they *need*. For many parents this is instinctual, but depending on the extent of your own childhood trauma, it may not be. If it is not, practical guidance can be found in *The Attachment Parenting Book: A Commonsense Guide to Understanding and Nurturing Your Child* by pediatrician William Sears, M.D. and childbirth educator and lactation consultant Martha Sears, R.N.

As the energetic disruptions from our childhood traumas heal, the resulting increase in consciousness frees us up to parent based on our understanding of our child's needs, not from our wounds. Such parental responsiveness to the needs of children fosters mutual respect and trust and creates secure attachment.

Adults affected by attachment trauma in their childhood experience difficulty in parenting the next generation in a number of ways. Less than a third of mothers who have attachment trauma themselves are able to securely attach to their own children, perpetuating the cycle of attachment trauma. Actress and author Tori Spelling poignantly conveys the anguish of insecure attachment trauma in her memoirs *Stori Telling* and *Mommywood*, relating her long and painful struggle to connect with her mother. Of the difficulty she faced overcoming this primary trauma in her own parenting, Spelling writes, "But knowing you want to do things differently doesn't mean you know how to escape the way you were raised."

Mothers who seek to fulfill their children's needs for attachment without having received it themselves can feel drained and emotionally exhausted. By attempting to meet their children's needs without having had their own needs met, they can in effect sacrifice their energy and themselves.

On the other hand, some adults who lack the vital experience of early dependence due to insecure attachment trauma become "helicopter parents," a term coined by Foster W. Cline, M.D. and Jim Fay with the 1990 publication of *Parenting With Love and Logic: Teaching Children Responsibility.* These "hovering" type of parents seek to control and remove all obstacles from their children's lives, which inadvertently prevents their children from experiencing the consequences of their actions and achieving independence.

When one has been traumatized in childhood, the impulse to protect one's own children from trauma is natural. However, children would be better served by parents who attend to their *own* unmet dependency needs, rather than projecting those unmet needs onto their offspring, sometimes well beyond childhood. In recent years parents have been known to intervene on their child's behalf with college administrators and human resource departments—negotiating grades, salaries, and promotions for their adult children.

Those with insecure attachment trauma can also project

their unmet dependency needs onto their pets. Although millions of cats and dogs in the U.S. are abandoned and mistreated, there are equal numbers who are pampered to the point of neurosis in households that lack clear boundaries or rules.

The answer to these parenting dilemmas created by attachment issues lies in breaking the cycle of trauma through the healing of unmet needs of both parents and children, a subject that will be discussed in chapter 10.

Why is it important to know about attachment trauma and its root causes? Because individuals who were insecurely attached to their parents feel unlovable and have difficulty accepting themselves as they are, a situation that *dramatically disrupts* our energy fields, similar to what happens when you reverse batteries in a battery-operated device—the current cannot flow and the device will simply not work. The same is true for our energy systems. When energy flow is not in alignment, it creates energetic resistance that is reflected in resistant behavior and health issues.

A state of self-rejection creates a strong block to healing through the dramatic disruption of energy flow created by energetic *reversal*. Energetic reversal is almost always present in chronic physical, emotional, mental, and spiritual conditions—such as addictions, depression, learning difficulties, weight issues, writer's block, athletic performance issues, and degenerative health conditions, such as cancer, multiple sclerosis, fibromyalgia, diabetes, arthritis, and auto-immune conditions.

When energy flow is disrupted from lack of acceptance, we are blocked from what we want most in our lives. When we don't accept ourselves as we are, our energy flow is not aligned with our desires, and we are working against ourselves. The wording of the affirmations at the end of each chapter in this book is designed to correct energetic reversal, especially when spoken while finger-tapping on the acupoints depicted in the appendix. More information on correcting energetic reversal through self-acceptance will be discussed in chapter 8.

Far-Reaching Effects

Attachment trauma has other far-reaching effects on health. The association between a childhood lacking a secure attachment to mother and a craving for sweets has been well-documented. It is no coincidence that Americans consume on average three to five pounds of sugar a week, as well as excess grains which the body converts to sugar, and alcohol, which is made from fermented grains and sugars. The consumption of excess sugar and grains disturbs pH balance, suppresses immune system function, and has been implicated in many of the major health issues facing Westerners today, such as cancer, diabetes, obesity, osteoporosis, heart disease, chronic fatigue, and depression. Alcohol abuse is associated with accidental injury, miscarriage, birth defects, relationship issues, anxiety, depression, cancer, and neurological, heart, liver, pancreas, and stomach issues.

Healing this national compulsion for sugars involves fulfilling our need for unconditional acceptance, which will be addressed in chapter 8—not by substituting the artificial sweetener aspartame for sugar. Researchers have found aspartame to be highly toxic, broken down by the body into formaldehyde and linked to the formation of brain tumors in consumers, as documented in the film *Sweet Misery* by Cori Brackett, who was a victim of aspartame poisoning.

Other health issues result from the emphasis in our society on instilling independence at too early an age. From the day a baby is born in the West, it seems the race is on for the child to sleep through the night, be weaned and eating independently, and become potty trained at the youngest possible age. When our natural individual developmental timeline is not respected and we are pushed to become independent at too early an age, we don't feel loved and accepted unconditionally, and can spend the rest of our lives arrested in this state of searching for that missing love, unable to "bloom" and experience interdependence, or proceed on the path to enlightenment that fully activates kundalini energy and opens our energy centers.

Unfortunately, this emphasis on early independence between mother and child contributes to low rates of breastfeeding, increased usage of artificial baby milk ("formula"), and early introduction of solid food, all of which cause immune system dysfunction that can persist throughout the lifespan in the form of food allergies, chronic infections, cancer, and autoimmune diseases. These negative health impacts are the unfortunate secondary consequences of Newtonian influences.

The prevalence of attachment trauma in our society may seem discouraging. But if we know that the pervasive issues suffered by those with attachment trauma is caused by a lack of unconditional love, then we know how to heal it—through unconditionally loving ourselves.

In the next chapter, we will look at other traumas and their energetic effect. Many of my clients believe that traumatic events in their past have no effect on their present state of health and well-being. But as we have seen....they do.

Even though I don't like to talk about or think about unpleasant occurrences from the past, I love and accept myself unconditionally, including my resistance.

Even though I may be afraid to let love in because I don't think I'm allowed, don't think I deserve it, or love has been hurtful in the past—I send love to every part of my subtle body and every cell of my physical body, including the parts of me that have been blocking love.

~7~

TRAUMA ENERGETICS

*"Trauma is a fact of life. It does not, however, have to
be a life sentence. Not only can trauma be healed,
but with appropriate guidance and support, it can
be transformative."*

—PETER LEVINE, PH.D.

"MY GRANDFATHER touched me inappropriately when
I was a child, but I've had counseling for that. I forgave him
a long time ago and let it go," said Helen in response to my
question about any history of childhood trauma. But while
Helen was telling me that this abuse and its aftermath were
behind her, her compromised energy and health picture were
telling me something entirely different. Although she had
mentally processed the past, her energy systems remained
disrupted, as reflected in her fertility issues, her sadness, and
her high degree of body tension. Complete healing had not
yet occurred.

In chapter 5 we looked at several examples of how sexual trauma affects energy systems; disrupting energy flow in the energy centers and meridians, and distorting the energy field. Like individuals affected by attachment trauma, survivors of sexual trauma usually lack self-acceptance and can carry guilt and shame. The child's psyche can interpret these "bad" experiences as meaning that *they* are bad. As we have learned, a state of self-rejection can dramatically disrupt the flow of energy in the human energy field, and guilt and shame states are associated with significantly diminished energetic frequency that is incompatible with health.

These disruptions in energy systems and energetic vitality can cause any number of physical, emotional, mental, and spiritual symptoms. The multitude of signs of sexual abuse are often missed or overlooked. These include memory difficulties, relationship issues, low self-esteem, panic attacks, anxiety, phobias, depression, trust issues, alcohol and drug abuse, obsessions and compulsions, nightmares, insomnia, suicidal thoughts, rage, emotional numbing, mood swings, arthritis, ADD, ADHD, headaches and migraines, eating disorders, PMS, chronic low back pain, gynecological and gastrointestinal issues, MS, chronic fatigue, fibromyalgia, lupus, self-injurious behavior, cancer of the reproductive structures and organs, and sexual dysfunction.

Although exact figures are unknown, and statistics undergo periodic modification to reflect new studies, the most current data indicates that one in three women and one in five men in the U.S. were sexually traumatized during childhood, clearly an epidemic situation. About half of those affected are initially unaware of their trauma due to unconscious memory suppression. In *The Sexual Healing Journey: A Guide for Survivors of Sexual Abuse,* licensed clinical social worker and sex therapist Wendy Maltz writes, "It is often not until survivors feel supported and secure that they begin to recall their sexual abuse."

Unfortunately this prevalence of disassociation and memory difficulties associated with sexual trauma has created tragic situations of false accusations. These false accusations of abuse against the innocent, which studies indicate occur in about 10 percent of cases, can instill doubt in the 90 percent who were genuinely victimized. In some situations, the "who, what, where, and when" of sexual trauma may never be entirely known. However, if we focus on any distressing symptoms and the disturbances in energy that are causing them in an unconditional way, deep healing can occur.

Many of the sexually traumatized clients I have worked with have been aware of their trauma, but some have not. And so, upfront, I want to say a word here about repressed memories related to childhood sexual trauma.

The media has sensationalized instances of therapist-planted, post-hypnotic suggestions of sexual trauma. Despite the fact that these cases have been magnified in the media, "forgotten" sexual trauma is very real. These cases where false charges have been trumped up make it unfortunate for those whose memory of sexual trauma has been repressed. I tread very lightly when I encounter indications that sexual trauma has occurred, and often avoid telling the client, to steer clear of unduly influencing them.

Whether or not I share the intuitive information I receive regarding sexual trauma requires careful consideration of the individual client, and then only with the understanding that such information should be considered within the context of all available information. My role as an energy medicine therapist is to work with the disruptions in energy systems that result from trauma, guided by my intuition—not to diagnose or provide proof of trauma. Survivors of sexual trauma usually also require the services of a psychotherapist with expertise in that area.

While working with Vanessa, during an information download from the universal energy field, I was shown images of sexual trauma she experienced as an infant. Although she had no conscious memory of this early traumatic event, her body receptors transmitted memories of the incident during the session in the form of uncomfortable sensations of pressure on her entire body and difficulty breathing, as if someone were lying on top of her. Vanessa also expressed emotional distress in the form of profound confusion.

Although the images I received from the incident were useful, the information was not necessary for me to assist Vanessa, nor did she need to remember what happened in order for the disturbances in her energy systems to release and be healed. In an atmosphere of trust, her energy systems automatically transmitted body memories for healing. By allowing her subtle and physical body to express what it was ready to without trying to control it, the energy disturbance was released.

Some clients I have worked with who do have intact memories of inappropriately sexualized situations in childhood may not recognize that they have been traumatized because there was no violence or force involved, they weren't physically hurt or threatened, or they didn't feel fear. Like Vanessa, they may have felt confused more than anything. Or, as with Helen, they may think that once the incident has been discussed with a counselor it is no longer an issue.

Any situation where the intention of an interaction with a child is sexualized, whether the child was exposed to adult body parts or sexual images with the intention to arouse, whether physical contact was implied or actual, and regardless of whether that contact was touch or actual penetration—all these scenarios can create trauma in the disrupting of energy systems that occurs, even when there is no awareness of the trauma. What's at issue is the violation of a delicate and important natural boundary in a child's consciousness. Overexposure, too soon, can result in trauma.

Western Medicine Trauma

Sometimes the very system that we turn to for healing the health issues that result from trauma-induced energy disruptions can itself be associated with trauma. The Western medical system can be a source of trauma for both consumers and providers. I have worked with many individuals who have come to me for healing after traumatic experiences with the allopathic community.

Conventional medical treatment can be painful and invasive, which is especially problematic for someone with a prior history of abuse. Surgical interventions disrupt the integrity of our physical and subtle bodies, the human energy field and energy systems. This trauma can be compounded if the invasive interventions prove ineffective.

People believe they have to subject themselves to uncomfortable, intrusive treatment that views their body as a biochemically driven machine for a variety of reasons. Either they are unaware of the nature of their bodies as energy and lack an understanding of the healing process, or they believe there isn't any other choice. Sometimes Western medicine *is* the best choice, especially in cases of acute or life-threatening illness or injury, but the point is—there should *be* a choice.

There is validity to feeling you don't have a choice in

healthcare. In the U.S., healthcare choices are severely limited in many areas by state laws that restrict the practice of natural healthcare. Healthcare choices have been limited by legal wars waged against effective herbal, nutritional, and immunological treatments for cancer, under the guise of protecting the public. In *When Healing Becomes a Crime: The Amazing Story of the Hoxsey Cancer Clinics and the Return of Alternative Therapies,* filmmaker and investigative journalist Kenny Ausubel exposes the failure of the "war on cancer." Ausubel tells the story of how the highly successful Hoxsey herbal treatment clinic was eventually blocked from operating in the U.S. In the film *Dying to Have Known,* filmmaker Steve Kroschel documents the negative campaign effectively waged against Gerson therapy, a proven nutritional program for cancer and other illnesses that can be found in *The Gerson Therapy,* by Charlotte Gerson and Morton Walker.

Most alarming is the lack of legal rights for U.S. parents to make the safest and most effective healthcare choices for their children. The documentary *Cut Poison Burn* chronicles the case of Thomas Navarro, who died as a direct result of mandated chemotherapy treatments that carried a high risk of injury and death, had little chance of success, and left his family bankrupt. His parents were legally coerced into conventional treatment through charges of child abuse and medical neglect, and blocked from using highly successful nontoxic antineoplastin treatment until *after* allopathy had failed, too late for Thomas.

Although many effective natural therapies for cancer are no longer available in the United States, some U.S. cancer treatment clinics have begun to offer nutritional and naturopathic therapy, but primarily as support for invasive surgery and toxic drug treatment. Although biochemical drugs and surgical treatment do not address the root cause of cancer, these treatments can delay death long enough to address the underlying energy imbalances associated with cancer. Researchers have made a clear connection between cancer and emotional repression and suppression, which create disturbances in energy.

The legal mandates for use of allopathy extend to medical professionals. Conventional medical doctors can suffer severe penalties for any deviation from established standards of Western medical practice, including loss of licensure. One physician I interviewed regarding nonconventional healing methods, whose story follows later in this chapter under the name of Dr. X, expressed great concern that his identity not be revealed, out of fear of those repercussions.

Consumer Trauma

"The physician acted like *he* was responsible for *my* health, and scolded me like a child when I didn't agree with his treatment plan," said Brooke, after a traumatic encounter.

For Rita, not feeling heard and having her distressing symptoms disregarded after a recent panic attack left her deeply traumatized. "None of the physicians I have consulted have listened to what I am saying. I literally couldn't breathe, and yet my symptoms were dismissed and the nurses treated me like that I was crazy. I've never felt so frightened and alone in my life. Tell me honestly, do you think I'm *crazy*?" she asked.

"My psychotherapist told me I was stupid and my ideas were dumb. I tried not to let it bother me, but I was crushed," said Vanessa.

These expressions of powerlessness and self-doubt after an encounter with a Western healthcare professional are not uncommon. When physical, emotional or mental distress is dismissed, when the focus is on the illness or disease and not the person, when our intuition is devalued and when separations are imposed between our physical, emotional, mental, and spiritual selves—trauma occurs.

Why is it so important to heal from medical trauma? Because medical trauma can result in either overuse or avoidance of Western medicine, both of which can have significant health consequences. Once victimized, consumers can become entrenched in victim consciousness and continue the pattern through repeated unnecessary invasive procedures. On the other hand, avoidance of Western medicine can prevent us from getting care that is necessary. Healing from being victims of medical trauma is about taking back our power to make our own health choices, and using Western medical professionals as consultants rather than figures who have authority over our health.

It is also important to understand why some allopathic professionals treat consumers in a way that traumatizes. They are a product of the Western culture they were raised in and many have suffered trauma in their own lives and in their training from which they have not recovered.

Provider Trauma

In *From Doctor to Healer: The Transformative Journey*, authors Robbie David-Floyd, Ph.D., medical anthropologist, and Gloria St. John, hospital administrator, have documented the traumatic experiences of many medical students. Like training for the armed forces, Western medical schools employ hazing techniques to break down the belief systems of initiates to prepare them for indoctrination into the "technomedical" model, achieved through a program of physical exhaustion from extreme overwork and cognitive overload from huge quantities of irrelevant material.

Many students enter medical school in the West with humanitarian goals, only to become cynical in a system they describe as "soul destroying" that emphasizes detachment and ignores the importance of self-reflection, intuition, and empathy. In *The Healing Power of Sound: Recovery from Life-Threatening Illness Using Sound, Voice, and Music,* oncologist Mitchell Gaynor, M.D. describes his "frustration verging on despair" with a medical system that failed to recognize the emotional needs of its consumers. Of his difficulties, Dr. Gaynor writes, "Every day I struggled with a medical culture that insisted I keep my distance from patients, and my inclination to get more deeply involved with them."

In Western medical school, basic sciences are taught in the Newtonian tradition, disconnected from any practical usage, an unintegrated approach that creates brain function imbalance—exaggerating left-brained, linear focus and creating narrow-mindedness. David-Floyd and St. John quote one unidentified physician: "It is only the most unusual individual who comes through a residency program as anything less than a technological clone."

Why does it matter how conventional medical professionals are trained? Because in our society, they have been the ones in charge of instructing us in how to care for our health. But how can providers help others if they haven't healed from their own traumatic experiences? How can a physician work with an individual in a holistic manner in a system that allocates only five to seven minutes for an office visit? How can a nurse provide holistic care in severely understaffed, task-oriented settings? And how can healthcare professionals teach us how to take care of ourselves when they have been trained to suppress their emotions and lead unhealthy, unbalanced lives? The answer to all these questions is the same: healing is greatly needed in our system of Western medicine.

Catalyst for Change

I have had similar experiences of trauma as both a consumer and provider of Western medical care. In a profession built on the principles of caring and compassion, I experienced little of either in nursing school, or in the clinical settings I worked in. Rather, I experienced judgment, criticism, and rejection from authority figures when I was at my most vulnerable—adding layers to energy blockages already present from childhood traumas. It was through the process of healing that I would see these experiences in a new light, a process that will be detailed in later chapters.

While the physician I consulted for infertility treatment was kind, caring, and concerned enough about my emotional well-being to refer me to a traditional talk therapist, the therapy was narrowly focused on managing the stress of the treatment—not on healing.

My physician's approach to infertility was limited to a search for pathology in the reproductive system, followed by expensive prescription drugs that had serious side effects and proved largely ineffective in facilitating a pregnancy. Likely the most frustrating aspect of allopathic infertility treatment, even more frustrating than my inability to conceive, was being treated like I was nothing more than my reproductive organs, as if they functioned independently and in isolation from the rest of my physical body, and separately from my emotional, mental, and spiritual selves. This created feelings of disintegration at a time when I most needed to feel whole.

Out of my deep desire to become a mother, I asked for and willingly subjected myself to this testing and treatment, because I didn't know any other way. But until my energy systems healed and I followed my intuition in the use of allopathic treatment as only one facet in a program of holistic care, I would not find success in completing our family.

As a clinical nurse working in a hospital setting, being forced to work in a fragmented, linear way in understaffed conditions made it impossible for me to provide the care that I knew my patients deserved. This energy-disrupting situation resulted in headaches and stomach pain.

In response to decreased reimbursement from health insurance companies, the administration of the hospital I worked for cut costs by doubling the number of patients each nurse on my unit cared for. By breaking down our shift literally minute-by-minute, and task-by-task, unit administration diagramed how we would care for twice as many patients in the same amount of time. Seeing my life's work reduced to a pile of checklists made me feel more like a factory worker than a nurse.

Although these traumatic experiences may seem negative and pointless, they can serve as *catalysts* for healing and transformation. Anything that increases the rate of a process is considered a catalyst, whether in reference to a chemical process or the healing process. When working environments become intolerable, when relationships fall apart, when we experience a health crisis, and when we have traumatic encounters with others—each can serve as a catalyst in that they accelerate healing. These situations are the workings of our deeper selves, attracting exactly the experiences we need to heal. We are not helpless victims to random life traumas. Our soul is in the driver's seat.

While practicing as a clinical nurse, I grew alarmed over the health of my colleagues. Many of the nurses I worked with suffered from debilitating health conditions, depression and general unhappiness; issues that I had also struggled with. In their eyes I saw my future. And with that awareness, the path seemed clear. I made the choice to gain knowledge and experience in energy medicine to help myself and others to create a different future.

For some physicians interviewed in *From Doctor to Healer*, a major life crisis such as illness or divorce created the opening for a paradigm shift. For others, the realization that their work was not helping people inspired change. For me, it was both.

Trauma as Catalyst

My disillusionment with Western medicine as both a consumer and provider served as the catalyst to pursue healing therapies and change the way I practiced nursing. Physicians who have successfully transitioned to practice holistically have had similar experiences. After healing from medical school trauma, Dr. Mitchell Gaynor was inspired to incorporate sound energy therapies into his oncology practice. After experiencing consumer trauma, Rita began a number of initiatives to help others, including leading support groups. Consumer trauma can also serve to shift health belief paradigms and prompt learning about, and seeking treatment for, the subtle body.

"The way I practice now began with this discovery about the retirement program for the internal medicine group practice I was in at that time," said Dr X, a physician I interviewed regarding his catalyst story. "While I was familiarizing myself with the retirement program, I realized that by my calculations, the group could not remain financially solvent while paying out such generous retirement benefits. So I kept asking questions and digging until I found out the benefits were based on age of death statistics for the physicians in the group. I was told that 35 percent to 40 percent of the physicians *were not expected to live to retirement age.*

"It seemed the physicians in the group practice were dying prematurely due to some unknown aspect of working with sick individuals on a daily basis. And this unknown aspect was having an ultimately fatal effect on the physicians themselves. I was determined to find out what this unknown aspect was, before I succumbed to it as well."

When a massage therapist effectively treated Dr. X's muscle strain with an energy healing technique, he was intrigued. "After the experience with the massage therapist, I started exploring energy healing, and I became convinced that sick people had 'sick' energy, and when healthcare workers interact with this toxic energy without healthy boundaries, the consequences can be premature death. I had found my unknown aspect."

Both energy medicine professionals and Western medical professionals face risks to self in daily work with the toxic energy fields of clients. Like the physicians in Dr. X's group practice, several healing practitioners in my local community have also died prematurely. Given this, anyone working in healthcare would be well-served by knowledge of the care of the subtle body. Knowing how to recognize the signs of toxic disturbances in one's energy systems and how to detoxify and heal those energetic disruptions is vital to health. In chapter 14, we will examine many everyday practices that can keep our vibrational levels high and energy fields clear.

Similar to my own experience, Dr. X did not accept energy

healing therapies at face value. He conducted his own personal research by becoming a consumer of many different energy-based modalities, and began studying to practice these therapies. Eventually Dr. X left his group internal medicine practice and started a new holistic medicine practice where he was in control of how much time he spent with clients. His new practice allowed time for his own self-care and the ability to integrate energy healing techniques in his work, although only with clients who signed a waiver.

Past Life Trauma

There is another category of trauma that may be a stretch for Western readers—especially those of the Christian faith—but warrants inclusion here. In Eastern traditions, the soul is considered timeless, and it is believed that we incarnate from one form to another. This belief is supported by a principle of physics called *the law of conversation of energy*, which states that energy may neither be created nor destroyed. According to this law, energy is never lost, but simply changes form.

As we are made of energy, Eastern religions theorize that the essence of who we are is never lost, but rather changes form from one lifetime to another. In the West, about half the population does not believe in the concept of reincarnation. The rest are divided between those who believe, and those who aren't sure.

As we learned in chapter 3, research findings indicate that memory is stored not in the brain, but in the universal energy field. If we accept these findings, along with the law of conservation of energy—then it becomes plausible that even after our physical bodies die, we continue in another form, and our memories remain in the field. This helps explain the widespread reporting of near-death experiences, and how those with high coherence with the field are able to access what appear to be memories from past lives and information about a person who has passed.

Evidence that cells continue to transmit memories after death lies in the recorded experiences of recipients of transplanted organs. In *The Heart's Code: Tapping the Wisdom and Power of Our Heart Energy*, neuropsychologist Paul Pearsall presents numerous cases in which transplant recipients demonstrated new knowledge and memories after surgery that were specific to the deceased donor of the transplanted organ they received.

Whether or not you believe in the existence of an "enduring self," some patterns that deeply influence our beliefs and behavior cannot be traced to any specific traumatic event in our lifetime. Even if we are able to relate a belief or pattern to a known trauma, that pattern of trauma may have begun in a prior life. Likewise, when we heal that pattern in this lifetime, it is said to heal in all others.

These vibrational patterns that leave an imprint on our consciousness from experiences in the past until they are healed are called *samskaras* in the East. The soul identification with these patterns is referred to as *karma*.

"Our beliefs, behavior, and energy patterns are unconsciously generated and shaped by these samskara vibrations," says Dr. John Wyrick, a former chiropractor and self-described "karmic doctor" who has been studying these patterns that vibrate in our energy fields for over 30 years. Dr. Wyrick has developed an effective method for ceasing the negative vibrational patterns that limit us, thus allowing positive karmic patterns to fully express. He calls his technique, "Nirodha Karma Healing," and has used this modality on thousands of individuals, often with stunning results.

To give you some examples, an individual with a wounded warrior pattern would likely have a tendency to feel anxious about their surroundings, and have a need to quickly categorize people they meet as friend or foe, even if they have never fought in a war. A person with an orphan pattern would be inclined to believe they have to do everything on their own and can't depend on others, even if supportive people are available in their life.

It is important to note that these karmic patterns are not conscious choices. As soon as you are born you begin vibrating in patterns such as rejection, victim, or betrayal. We carry these patterns from lifetime to lifetime, until they are healed. Depending on which patterns you vibrate in, you attract experiences that vibrationally match those patterns. So we see that karma is not about what we deserve, or about punishment. Rather, karmic patterns govern what we attract, which is unconscious.

In my own work, I have found that when I correctly identify a karmic pattern that is currently impacting a client, their energy system will respond strongly. For example, when I intuitively used the words "trauma from untimely death" while tapping Rita's acupoints, she felt a wave of energy that left her entire body tingling and buzzing. "I've never felt anything like that," she said. "I really resonated with those words, which is strange, because obviously I haven't died. Although I have to admit that when I have really bad panic attacks, I feel like I'm going to die."

Trauma *DOES NOT MEAN* Drama

"I hate to use the word trauma, because it sounds so dramatic, but I have to admit that the circumstances surrounding my daughter's months in the intensive care nursery still distress me," said Whitney. Like many of my clients, Whitney was reluctant to use the word trauma because of the misunderstanding that trauma must include drama.

I hear statements such as this frequently in my interactions with clients—the tendency to discount past experiences, and the difficulty recognizing trauma, even when distress from past experiences is clearly present.

While some of the traumas I have discussed in this book are indeed dramatic in nature, drama is not a requirement for trauma. Trauma comes in all shapes and sizes. What defines trauma is not the *nature* of the event, but its *impact* on energy systems. What is traumatic for one person does not necessarily cause trauma for another. If it is distressing to you, it doesn't matter whether it would be distressing for someone else. All emotional responses are valid.

An event that may seem of little consequence at the time can be traumatic in that it creates significant energetic disruption. If our energy systems are already disrupted by earlier trauma, how we respond to future events is compromised. Although a securely attached person may respond to an event like just a bump in the road of life, an insecurely attached person may experience major disruption.

In a later session with Steven, he shared that he had been recently feeling a lot of anger toward his father, and he wasn't sure what it was about. While he lay on my healing table, I connected with him in the energy of unconditional acceptance—listening to his rhythms without judgment. In that supportive energy he had a spontaneous memory from a childhood event that seemed trivial on the surface, yet had altered the course of his life.

At the age of six, Steven's father attempted to teach him how to ride a bike. The first time his father let go of the bike, Steven fell and began crying, prompting his father to abruptly end the lesson. When Steven was never offered another bike-riding lesson, he felt his father had given up on him. Lacking the skill of riding a bike, he felt different and separated from others, unable to participate in riding events with friends and family, even into adulthood.

From this early experience grew a belief pattern that would rule Steven's existence—that he had to constantly keep "pedaling" through life alone because no one was going to help him, and if he lost his balance and fell, he would never get another chance to succeed. His "failure" to learn how to ride a bike reflected in a general feeling of inadequacy related to his body, a perspective that was eventually reflected in his bodily functioning.

In the next chapter, we will examine how trauma shapes beliefs, and how we tend to suppress our emotional responses. As we shall see, this creates a fundamental problem because emotion is the *language* that we use to communicate with the universal energy field.

Even though I may have been reluctant to recognize trauma in my life, and minimized its presence, I completely love and accept myself, and recognize that whatever I am feeling is valid.

Even though traumatic experiences from the past may seem discouraging and pointless, I lovingly embrace myself in the knowledge that there are no mistakes, only healing opportunities.

~ 8 ~

ENERGETIC SUPPRESSION

*"Beliefs are vibrational forces that create
the physical basis for our individual lives and our health."*

—CHRISTIANE NORTHRUP, M.D.

AS I RELATED at the beginning of this book, my work has evolved from my own healing process that began over twenty years ago. Like many of my clients, I have experienced both attachment trauma and sexual trauma. From both personal and professional experience, I know firsthand some of the messages children perceive from these traumas:

- You are not loved or accepted unconditionally
- You are not worthy or valued
- You are not good enough
- You are damaged goods
- You are shameful
- You are not safe
- You cannot trust people

As I have mentioned before, the traumatic incidents at the root of these negative beliefs do not have to be remembered for energy disturbances to occur. The negative messages do not even have to be spoken to us to create disruption. We communicate through energy, conveyed through the intention of our actions. For example, a pre-verbal child innately senses the difference between a touch in their best interests, such as a parent bathing them or a health care professional examining them, and a touch with a different intention, as in a touch with sexual overtones—even if these touches feel kinesthetically identical and involve the same part of the body.

Although the child may not cognitively understand the difference between these touches, they know that one makes them feel good, cared for, and accepted, while the other makes them feel bad, confused, or anxious—the result of energy disruption. These messages are conveyed through energy and form our belief systems, creating pervasive feelings of low self-worth and low self-esteem.

The energetic disruption caused by trauma produces low energetic frequency states, such as shame, guilt, apathy, grief, fear, desire, anger, and pride. These states are associated with negative belief systems and a sense of powerlessness. And the powerlessness that these low energy states create is associated with the use of force—forceful self-rejecting thoughts and forceful treatments. The use of force in traumatized individuals can actually prevent them from healing and recovering. In this chapter and others, we will be exploring this association between low energy frequency states, powerlessness, and the use of force against ourselves and others.

It's important to look at our beliefs because every cell of our bodies responds to the energetic frequency of those beliefs. Our beliefs become a program that our body runs on moment-to-moment, whether positive or negative.

Other traumas experienced in childhood that also impact our self concepts include:

- disabilities
- illness
- injuries
- bullying
- accidents
- natural disasters
- exposure to violence or violent images

The man who was born with abnormalities in his urinary system that resulted in chronic infections developed a deep-seated belief that he was broken and a "freak," despite having an otherwise secure, loving childhood.

After Brooke's car accident, she developed a global belief that the world was not safe, and that danger loomed around every corner.

After Steven fell off his bike as a child during his first and only riding lesson, he formed a belief that if he cried he would be abandoned, so he decided never to cry again. A single fall from a bicycle usually wouldn't be considered trauma, but when we look at the situation holistically, we can see how that incident fits in the larger picture.

"I never felt close to my mother," said Steven. "She was emotionally unavailable. From a very young age, I felt like I had to be completely independent, because I couldn't rely on anyone."

The trauma of insecure attachment to his mother, and the beliefs he formed as a result, impacted his ability to process the trauma of his fianceé's death, as well as his ability to reach out for help.

"I never cried when she was killed, my fianceé," Steven added.

"Did you receive any professional assistance after she died?" I asked.

"Not until now," he said. "I never connected what happened with the health problems I was having. She died so long ago, and I assumed my problems were simply the result of aging."

This is a widely held cultural belief, that aches, pains and diminished body functioning are an inevitable consequence of aging, rather than the effect of a lifetime of unaddressed, accumulated trauma on energy systems.

Steven—based on his belief that crying causes abandonment—suppressed his emotions, which I had perceived in his first session as a jangly sensation in his energy rhythms. And the act of trying to constantly stay upright on that metaphorical bicycle of life had meant driving himself to exhaustion in his work. The decision he made at a young age motivated by self-preservation predisposed him to suppress the emotional effects of the trauma when his fianceé was killed.

Beliefs Form Energy Blocks

I would like to share my experience of disturbed energy flow while writing these chapters—a blockage in energy that stemmed from my own negative beliefs. Each time I attempted to write about how energy blockages are formed, information from my unconscious mind would flood my conscious mind. Like doing a search on the Internet, my mind would go in many different directions at once, all interconnected. The difficulty of finding a straight path through a web of information would make my shoulders and neck muscles tight, and cause headaches that repeatedly forced me to stop writing. But there was more to it, something beneath the frustration.

I finally let go of even trying to write. I closed my eyes and focused instead on taking some slow, deep breaths, and shifted into a meditative state. In an instant, words came to me –*You can't do this because you are stupid and have no common sense.*

It all came back in a flash. These were words I frequently heard as a child, my father's criticism. Regardless of whether that judgment was an expression of his own low self-worth, those words had traumatized me, and that trauma created the unconscious belief that I am not smart enough to write a book. My symptoms indicated an energy disruption created by the trauma and the belief that formed from that trauma. With this belief now conscious, I had two choices. I could continue judging myself as not smart enough, or I could accept every part of myself unconditionally. All too often we choose the former, because we don't know any other way.

The flow of writing had to come *through* me, not *from* me, and as long as this belief about my intelligence remained, that flow was blocked. By using some of the energy medicine practices detailed in chapter 14, I was able to release the energy blockage caused by my father's judgment, which had created the negative belief about myself and the headaches.

We have explored how the traumas of our lives result in negative beliefs. Now let's look at the next step in the formation of energy blockages, self-judgment and criticism, and the role of suppression in more detail.

Disturbances in energy occur when traumatic experiences become forcefully *suppressed* due to a variety of factors, such as cultural socialization, ideology, and belief systems. Let's examine these one at a time.

The Western Culture of Suppression

Even if you are free of any significant childhood trauma, if you grew up in the West, you likely have issues of suppression, or non-acceptance, although I have worked with individuals who grew up in the East who have issues with suppression as well. Earlier, we explored some of the reasons suppression is so rampant in our culture—Newtonian-Cartesian influences that emphasize separatism over connectedness, and view the body as a machine.

In the West, the suppression of emotion is prized. We speak highly of those who don't show emotion. For example, appearing stoic at a funeral of a loved one is interpreted as "handling it well." The message is clear: holding it in is *good*, and letting it out is *bad*. But the consequences of "holding it all together" are disrupted energy flow, the precursor to illness and disease conditions.

Emotional suppression and body suppression go hand-in-hand. In *Discovering The Body's Wisdom,* massage therapist and holistic health expert Mirka Knaster writes, "We learned to hold back our fear and terror, our anger and rage, by tightening our muscles, keeping ourselves from crying or screaming, in order not to lose connection with a parent, or other caretaker, in order to win approval, acceptance, or love, or in order to survive."

Knaster outlines how families, communities, ethnic groups, religions, and educational systems have negatively influenced the formation of our self-image. Children are admonished for touching themselves, required to stand up straight, instructed to hold their legs together, and expected to sit rigidly at a desk all day. These childhood instructions and admonitions can cause us to suppress our bodies as a source of pleasure and a vehicle for expression of emotion. This suppression can continue throughout our life, until healing occurs.

Often we are not aware we are suppressing our bodies and our emotions. When suppression is unconscious, it is referred to as *repression*. Repression is a natural response that can occur when we do not feel unconditionally accepted in childhood.

Emotional suppression and repression are frequently at the root of impaired health that does not respond to allopathy. Even the conservative Center for Disease Control and Prevention estimates that 85 percent of diseases have an emotional basis.

When it comes to health, the Western mentality is warlike, with an emphasis on using force through "fighting" illness, "declaring war" on disease and "conquering" health issues. This battle against health issues is accomplished through suppressive drugs that eradicate symptoms—stamping out the vital messages from our body-mind that let us know when our energy is blocked or disrupted. When treatment for health issues is conducted like a military operation, our body-minds become a battlefield.

In addition to suppressing the messages from our bodies, the use of biochemical medication to treat energy blockages has other consequences. When suppressive medication is discontinued, suppressed symptoms can reappear in different and sometimes more dangerous forms. When the healing process is obstructed through suppressive treatment, symptoms can become chronic.

We can see this problem of suppressing symptoms in cases of inflammation. In naturopathic philosophy, inflammation is considered a necessary part of the healing process that occurs while the body processes waste material. When acute illness is allowed to express while being managed through natural means, it can be purifying in nature. If acute illness is suppressed and the underlying energetic blockage is not corrected; if the body's attempts to heal the condition are suppressed—eventually the body-mind can no longer overcome the condition and chronic illness results.

In the previous chapter, we considered the importance of achieving energy balance. In light of this, we can now see how suppressing symptoms can create chronic health conditions epidemic in the West. This treating of conditions from the "outside-in" runs contrary to principles of healing, which we will explore further in chapter 10.

The forceful war mentality seen in all aspects of Western culture, including healthcare, is also reflected in how we treat ourselves. When we draw inner lines of battle, pitting parts labeled as "good" against the parts labeled "bad," we create enemies within.

Why is it important to heal suppression? Because as long as we are in suppression, *trauma cannot resolve.* And unresolved trauma can negatively impact health and cause significant long-term anxiety and phobias, compulsions, obsessions, and addictions—all in an attempt to decrease the anxiety through suppression, avoidance, and control

Nora developed a phobia of driving on highways after her brother was killed in a high-speed car crash. She also began compulsively overeating and obsessively cleaning her house. Nora did not realize she was using food and cleaning to suppress and avoid anxiety, that her phobia was related to the trauma of losing her brother, or that her obsession was an attempt to regain control. We have seen how unresolved attachment trauma can cause an addiction to sugar. Unfortunately, engaging in compulsions and addictions to manage anxiety does not relieve the anxiety. It only covers it up. Addictions, epidemic in the U.S., are an unconscious attempt to suppress anxiety.

In our work together, Jim related that although he had been unhappy for most of his marriage, separating from his wife did not improve his situation. But even so, he was reluctant to explore the roots of his unhappiness in his troubled childhood. In time, Jim would realize that isolating himself from relationships was only a means of avoiding his feelings, another form of suppression.

Taught to Suppress

Suppression begins in the home. Parents may encourage their children to ignore their feelings or push them down, or to reject parts of themselves as they may have been taught to do in their childhood. Parents do this by example—by rejecting what they don't like in themselves, or by rejecting what they don't like to see in their children—because it reminds them of what they don't like in themselves... their shadow.

In a household where she was not heard or accepted as she was, Rita had tantrums of protest until she was five years old. She eventually gave up and attempted to become someone her parents would approve of. She was rewarded for becoming docile and compliant by being told she was "good." Now in her late 30s, she has pushed parts of herself that she has labeled "bad" so far down into the shadow—she doesn't even know who she really is.

Rita took over the job of parenting herself when she became an adult, and that included rejecting parts she didn't like, as her parents taught her. Like Rita, we play roles in the world to receive acceptance because we don't believe we can be loved just as we are. We think we have to conform and be inauthentic in order to "earn" love.

The "authentic" Rita is feisty and full of fire, but to her, those characteristics were unacceptable. In order to be acceptable, she developed a false, compliant ego self. The consequences of maintaining this false self were tension, anxiety, and debilitating insomnia.

As beliefs are energy, Rita's cells responded to her self-rejecting energy pattern by attacking itself in the form of Graves' disease, an autoimmune condition.

Some religious traditions encourage aligning ourselves with dogma and certain sets of acceptable behaviors. In order to comply, we reject the parts of us that are not aligned with this dogma—causing us to suppress or conceal other behaviors. This creates fracturing within ourselves.

In Rita's religion, only men are allowed to hold positions of power and are considered to have authority over women. This was another factor in her unconscious decision to become docile, compliant, and powerless. For Dennis, religious beliefs led him to bury a big part of himself, his sexual orientation, because it wasn't acceptable in his religion. Eventually he became disabled with rheumatoid arthritis, an autoimmune condition. We will read more about Dennis's story later in this chapter.

Parents can reject what they perceive as "dark" behavior in their child, or when they feel insecure about their children's abilities in relation to their own. For example, when Claire, the lady who felt constantly criticized, was a child, her father would make a point of comparing her cooking and piano playing with her mother's. When he commented that Claire could now play the piano better than her mother, his wife bristled. Soon Claire's mother got rid of the piano. She also talked Claire out of going to college because it would mean Claire would have more education than her. Claire developed a pattern of holding herself back in life and suppressing her natural talents.

We suppress aspects of ourselves that remind us of parts that we don't like in our parents or others. Rita rejected the parts of herself that reminded her of her parents. Seeing her mother's selfishness in her own behavior was so distressing, Rita rejected any part of her that she felt was selfish. Since stubbornness reminded her of her father, Rita rejected her stubbornness as well. As we worked together, she was surprised to experience physical pains as she became conscious of her self-rejection. How is physical pain related to emotions?

Emotional Suppression and Physical Pain

As you may recall from chapter 3, the practice and writings of musculoskeletal pain expert John Sarno, M.D., are based on his premise that the expression of emotional pain is so unacceptable in our society that we unconsciously choose to experience it as physical pain. As long as we are focused on physical pain, we remain "distracted" from the unacceptable emotions that are repressed. In *Healing Back Pain: The Mind-Body Connection*, Dr. Sarno writes, "What has been described is universal in our culture; only the degree of repressed emotionality varies. And in our culture, nature has created a mechanism whereby we can avoid being aware of those bad feelings—it gives us physical symptoms."

This unconscious desire to avoid emotional pain is so strong, once a particular ailment is recognized as an emotional problem in disguise, we will shift symptoms to a new ailment. This is the same phenomenon I have seen when working with clients—pain that suddenly moves to different areas of the body once it has been exposed. This movement from one condition to another can be seen en masse, culture-wide. We have gone from epidemic levels of headaches and gastrointestinal ailments reported in the 1970s, to chronic back, neck and shoulder pain, fibromyalgia, and carpal tunnel syndrome in more recent years. The bias against emotional problems is so strong, people have difficulty accepting that any of these conditions are emotionally based.

As noted by Dr. Sarno in *The Divided Mind,* the presence of bacteria in the gastrointestinal tracts of individuals with ulcers and irritable bowel syndrome only fueled the belief that these diseases are purely physical. As we know from naturopathic philosophy, pathogens are not the primary cause of disease but are the secondary effects of imbalances in our energy systems. It is also important to note that, regardless of whether one is only aware of the physical symptoms of the imbalance, the imbalance affects all levels—emotional, mental, spiritual, and physical. In other words, it is inaccurate to label any condition as only physical, only emotional, only mental, or only spiritual.

Physicians admittedly feel more comfortable treating ailments that present in the physical body, referring mental and emotional difficulties to psychiatrists for medication. However, mental and emotional difficulties are not separate issues—nor do biochemical medications "heal" emotional and mental distress; they suppress symptoms.

This bias against emotional issues extends to health insurance, which typically covers diagnostic testing and treatment for physical ailments, while excluding benefits for mental and emotional conditions. It is little wonder that we unconsciously choose physical pain over emotional pain.

Suppressing Emotions
During the years I worked in clinical nursing, I was concerned

about my patients' emotional well-being, but I didn't understand the role it played in health. Likewise, when I first began working as a healing practitioner, I didn't focus on emotions. Initially my sessions were quiet, other than an occasional question from the client or their rare spontaneous emotional outburst. Emotions, I thought, were "messy" and belonged in a psychotherapist's office. But it was apparent that I wasn't fully helping my clients get to the root of their issues.

Although clients in my practice did heal, that healing occurred much faster and on a much deeper level once I began connecting to their emotional state. And the more I began to explore their emotional states, the more I realized that helping them connect to their emotions was the key to gaining access to healing.

Like thoughts and beliefs, emotions are energy, and as such are meant to move through the body with the flow of energy. I'm sure you've had the experience of laughter or joy as it rippled through your body, leaving you tingly all over. It feels like a wave of energy, because it *is*. Believe it or not, even "negative" emotions such as grief can be experienced in the same manner.

Sadness and anger are just as valid as joy and happiness. You can't experience one and suppress the other. It doesn't work that way. By freezing out your sadness, you also freeze out happiness. If you shut out anger, you shut out joy and passion too. However, unpleasant feelings such as sadness, grief, anger, resentment, and loneliness are typically suppressed in an effort to prevent them from intensifying and spreading. But when we suppress our emotions, we obstruct the flow of our energy, and create a sense of separation from the universal energy field. The result is exhaustion and disconnection.

Let's face it. Most people don't like emotions, or at least what we consider "negative" emotions. We don't want to feel anger or sadness, and we certainly don't want to cry. We don't want to appear "weak" to others, and may fear that expressing our emotions may hurt those around us. Some people become angry with me when I suggest they take a look at their emotions, like Helen, who asked, "You aren't going to make me cry, are you?" Clients may shed some tears over the course of a session, but it is not my goal to "make" someone cry.

When clients do cry, they usually cover their face with their hands in shame and say, "I'm sorry." Because we are nearly universally uncomfortable with our emotions in our culture, my clients assume that showing emotion in my presence is going to make *me* uncomfortable as well. But the more we can be accepting of our own emotions, the easier it is to be accepting of the emotions of others.

For many, suppressing emotional distress creates a situation where we don't even know what we're feeling. When we are experiencing a disturbance in energy that creates emotional, physical, mental, or spiritual distress that we don't have words for, we call it *stress*. But as we discussed in chapter 3, what we refer to as stress is a reaction to a situation based on belief systems. Fear and worrying cause stress, but the question is—*what belief is causing the fear and worrying?*

Vanessa had an underlying belief that nothing she did was good enough. That belief created what she identified as "work stress," because no matter how diligently Vanessa went about her work, she did not believe she was doing a good enough job. The energetic frequency of her belief disrupted energy flow, creating distress in the form of muscle tension, anxiety, and an upset stomach, which she labeled as "stress."

When we suppress our emotions, it affects not only how we treat ourselves, but how we treat others. If we don't like our own emotions, it makes it difficult to react appropriately to the emotions of others. One of my clients related that days after his adult son's attempted suicide, friends urged him to move on. "I couldn't believe it. The message was—I'm not comfortable with your emotions, so stop talking about it so I won't be uncomfortable," he said. After Audrey's second miscarriage, if she mentioned her loss to a friend, they would respond with a story about someone who had lost a pregnancy at a later stage. "It was as if they were saying that I didn't have a right to grieve, because someone else had it worse than me. As if my loss did not matter as much as someone else's," said Audrey.

We fear that if we affirm the negative feelings of others, their emotions will escalate. But in fact, it's just the opposite. How often do we say "You shouldn't feel that way," "You have no reason to be upset," or "Look on the bright side," to those who share their emotional upset? These comments serve as messages of suppression. In effect they say to others—*how you feel is unacceptable*, which only compounds blockages in energy. Acknowledging with compassion where someone is emotionally actually defuses strong emotions and enhances energy flow.

I ask that you not criticize yourself if you have made these comments to others. Before I studied energy medicine, I said them as well. Expressions of suppression are nearly universal. The important thing is to know that the cycle of suppression can be broken through compassion for yourself and others. Compassionate validation creates connection and energy flow, whereas invalidation creates disconnection and energy blockages. Feeling is part of being human, and allowing the expression of emotions is what makes us feel *alive*.

Why is it so important to understand suppression? Because as we saw in chapter 5, suppression creates blocks in our energy systems, which result in health issues. For example, Tess developed arthritis when she suppressed her anger. And in chapter 7, the many distressing symptoms associated with sexual trauma were all caused by suppression of emotions. In later chapters we will hear other stories of emotional suppression causing health issues. However, it's not just our emotions that we suppress. We also suppress our sexuality, and even our negativity.

Suppressing Sexuality

Dennis grew up in a small community where "boys were boys and girls were girls."

"It was made very clear that any boy who had feelings for another boy was a 'fag.' And fags were boys who were hated and got beat up.

"That posed a serious problem for me," says Dennis, "because I knew by the time I was five that the older boys in the neighborhood attracted me in a much more powerful way than did the pretty girls. It was something I felt deep in my gut, physically, though not sexually of course at that age. But feeling the hatred and angry energy of the other boys scared the hell out of me."

So Dennis buried his feelings under layers of silence and shame. "The indirect but very strong message to me was: You're a twisted, hateful being, and you deserve to be beaten to a pulp."

Dennis was also brought up in a highly religious home, where sex and sexuality were never discussed. And when he reached high school he became involved in the Jesus Movement of the early 1970s, and became a devout Christian teenager. "One of the main reasons I made such a conscious move to be devout was, by the time I was 15 I hated myself. I wanted to commit suicide...but that was considered a 'mortal sin' and I was afraid I'd burn in hell forever. So I gave my life—and very secretly, my desire to be 'healed' of homosexuality—to Jesus. I fully expected to have this 'spiritual cancer' miraculously cut out of me."

Dennis did all the "right" things, according to his Christian training. He read the Bible, lead youth groups and Bible studies, sought help for his "besetting sin" from pastors and Christian counselors—and he got married. "I would not have done that without the counsel, direction, and blessing of my spiritual leaders, but they believed that was part of Jesus' 'cure.'"

And so Dennis married, and in a few years, became the father of three children. "I truly loved my wife. And I adored my three kids. They were my world. My life. I was utterly in love with and faithful to my wife and children. And I continued serving God through churches...but I also began to experience a lot of unexplainable sickness."

At first it was exhaustion. Then came the low-grade fevers and complete physical depletion. "I'd sleep for nine, ten, eleven hours, then wake up and barely be able to drag myself out of bed. When I jogged a mile I'd stress my immune system, and be down for the count for days with fevers and painfully swollen lymph glands throughout my body."

Years of pain and exhaustion dragged on. Test after medical test turned up nothing. "Physicians got tired of me coming back to them with the same problem—and they had no diagnosis. One told me not to come back for at least 18 months, 'or if you have a *real* problem we can deal with.'

"All the while I was experiencing mental and emotional stress, because I felt sexually attracted to men—but I would never entertain the thought of cheating on my wife or endangering her health or mine by acting out with someone and possibly introducing a sexually transmitted disease into either of our health pictures.

"And while I knew many national leaders of so-called ex-gay ministries, I also knew their 'success' rate in 'changing' people was extremely limited. At most they helped sex addicts to stop having non-stop sexual liaisons with multiple partners...that's about it. I met too many men and women who had been in these ministries for many years without changing one bit. So I knew there was no help for me there."

For years, the double weight of Dennis's denied sexuality and his shame at being gay, together with the weight of his physical ailments, dragged him further down into the dark. His health began to fail, and he fought—month after month, year after year—with suicidal depression. "And every day I was getting up, putting a happy Christian smile on my face, and going off to work, or to lead a Bible study. I was in hell."

After more than ten years of struggle, the bottom fell out—at least physically. One day, Dennis woke up with every joint in his body inflamed. His hands and feet were in tremendous pain, and his hips, shoulders, and knees were on fire.

The official diagnosis was rheumatoid arthritis—an autoimmune disorder—and one physician put him on a course of pharmaceuticals. "These were powerful drugs, but they didn't touch the pain. My hands became claws, and sometimes I could hardly walk. The depression and exhaustion were terrible—a nightmare."

After two more years of allopathic treatments, a new, consulting physician reviewed Dennis's charts, and after a physical exam, said, "I want to suggest something new."

Dennis was all ears.

"Autoimmune conditions like yours very often have a psychosomatic component, maybe even a basis," the new physician explained. "That doesn't mean you're crazy or you're imagining you're sick. It means you may have some deep-lying tension that is stressing your whole being. It's like a switch is left on, and you're burning up all your energy without being aware of it, depleting your body." Then came the clincher.

"If there is some emotional issue in your life that you need to face and deal with, I recommend that you do," the physician said. "Or this syndrome that has you will likely kill you."

"It was like being given the choice—'the devil? or the deep blue sea?' When I walked out of his office I knew *exactly* what I had to do in order to recover and live. And I wanted to for the sake of my kids. But I was also in agony at another level... because I knew that facing the fact that I was—I am—a gay man would mean ending my marriage. I broke down there in the parking lot for almost an hour before I could even drive.

"But that was the day my life changed *and* my healing began. In fact, once I made the tough, tough decision that I would have to own my true sexuality—a piece of my core identity—my symptoms began to lessen *immediately.* It would take me years to carefully redirect my family relationships—to divorce as painlessly as anyone who deeply loves another person can, and to guide my children through the big change—but the plain fact is this:

"Once the severe wound at the core of my being was healed when I accepted my sexual identity, *my physical energy returned immediately and my body healed in two weeks.*"

Dennis would go on to run marathons, triathlons, and even an ironman race, all in his late 40s. He remains pain- and symptom-free to this day, some ten years after his own personal identity and energy healing.

Many of my clients tell me that their physicians are up front about the fact that they have no idea what causes autoimmune diseases like the rheumatoid arthritis that devastated Dennis. The word autoimmune means "self attack." Simply put, autoimmune disease is associated with the energetic disruption of *self-rejection.* Regardless of how that rejection manifests in your physical body, and what Western medical diagnosis it has been labeled with— whether chronic fatigue syndrome, fibromyalgia, Hashimoto thryroiditis, Graves' disease, inflammatory bowel disease, Sjogren's syndrome, lupus, or rheumatoid arthritis—in my experience it is the energy of self-rejection that precedes disease symptoms. And as Dennis's story so clearly illustrates, it is the energy of *self-acceptance* that can reverse and heal these disease states.

Suppressing Negativity

Some people suppress and bury what they perceive as their negativity because they believe this is the path to thinking "positive."

Helen was a woman with a lot on her plate. She worked full-time as a business executive, managed the care of her elderly father, and had been pursuing treatment for infertility for years, unsuccessfully. After reading some self-help books about positive thinking, she felt strongly that staying positive was her path to healing. She believed that as long as she stayed positive the effects of being inappropriately touched as a child by her grandfather, as well as the effects of her current infertility, were negated.

When I asked Helen how she was feeling about her infertility, she said, "Fine. Peaceful." But I noticed there were tears welling up in her eyes, she was barely breathing, and her entire body appeared tense. With some gentle questioning, Helen revealed that she was indeed sad, and rated that sadness at a *nine* on a scale of one to ten, ten being the worst possible sadness. But despite that high self-rated sadness, she quickly dried her tears and re-stated that she was fine and peaceful, as if she were reading words off a cue card. "I don't want to talk about my sadness, OK? I've got to stay positive," said Helen.

Helen's desire to remain positive was understandable, but in denying her true feelings, it was difficult for me to help her. Her resistance kept her energy blockages in place. In the next chapter we will revisit Helen as we examine the steps of healing.

In my experience, positive thinking occurs naturally when negativity is allowed to fully express to completion without judgment. Deep healing *includes* exploring our "darkness." But beyond *thinking* positive, it's more important to *feel* positive. Why? Because science has shown us that it is through our emotions that we connect to the universal energy field.

The Science of Emotions

In Eastern traditions, emotions are said to arise from consciousness. In the Western view, emotions are thought to originate in the brain. Through breakthrough research conducted by Candace Pert, Ph.D., author of *The Molecules of Emotion*, we have a better understanding of the biochemical processes that produce the feeling of an emotion. However, research is only just beginning regarding the energy processes that *initiate* those biochemical processes. It is the *energy* of a thought that generates a biochemical response and the release of hormones which result in the *feeling* of an emotion such as joy, fear, anger, or sadness. As we know, that feeling can also be expressed physically. Thinking and feeling are the result of processing quantum information in the brain and body.

In the last twenty years, a number of experiments have shed light on the interaction of energy with our cells. In an experiment conducted by quantum biologists Vladimir Poponin and Peter Gariaev at the Russian Academy of Science, scattered photons of light energy in a vacuum responded to the presence of living DNA by arranging themselves in a pattern. In another experiment conducted by the U.S. Army, DNA taken from a subject responded *in sync* to the subject's emotional states by exhibiting a measureable, simultaneous electrical response, regardless of how many miles the subject was separated from their own cells. And in the final experiment cited here, researchers at the Institute of HeartMath found that DNA in a glass beaker changed its shape when exposed to focused, intentional emotion.

From these examples of ground-breaking experiments, we see how cells communicate through energy, particularly the energy of emotion. When we suppress our emotions, energetic communication is disrupted, affecting the systems of the subtle and physical body. Once suppressed emotions are released and energy flow and communication are restored, the body can do its biochemical repair work. Thus healing on an emotional level gives us access to healing on all levels.

We have completed our exploration of the steps in the creation of an energy blockage; trauma, beliefs, and suppression. But there is another aspect of the formation of energy blockages I have noted in my work that I would like to share with you, the concept of *layers*.

Layers of Impact

In previous chapters, we have seen how living in a state of blocked energy affects us over time. An initial energy blockage can become the foundation on which our beliefs, self-concepts, and identity are built. Layer upon layer, blockage by blockage, energy disturbances can be laid down over a lifetime.

The energy of trauma disrupts our natural rhythms, our energetic frequencies, and the very structure of our systems. With each new layer of energy-disrupting trauma, the overall vitality of the body-mind is further compromised, resulting in disease.

Regardless of whether one believes that traumatic experiences could have originated in this lifetime or previous ones, these experiences tend to become repeating patterns. As our energy fields have electromagnetic qualities with attraction properties, we tend to attract the same situations, over and over, until the pattern is broken.

Vanessa's pattern of hurt and disappointment originated in her childhood. She recalled numerous situations while growing up when her parents could have shown her that they loved and cared for her. When they consistently didn't, she felt deeply hurt. This pattern continued into adulthood, with a series of relationships with hurtful friends, creating layer upon layer of hurt.

Gary Craig, founder of Emotional Freedom Techniques, likens this to a diseased forest where each tree represents a specific negative event that compounds and deepens blockages to energy flow. Vanessa had a metaphorical "forest of hurt," containing a tree for each of the many times she had been hurt throughout her life. It was a forest that over time had become as thick and impassable as a jungle. Trapped inside this jungle, Vanessa was unable to find her way out until healing interventions thinned out her "forest," weakening the structure of energy blockages until they collapsed.

In my own situation, the first layer of trauma began in the first years of my life through insecure attachment and sexual trauma. Infant feeding practices that included early introduction of solid food coupled with the frequency of rejection resulted in food allergies and autoimmune disease. In turn, unbeknownst to the Western medical professionals I consulted, autoimmune disease was a key factor in my infertility. In another layer, I was traumatized by the Western medical infertility treatment itself. These traumas created negative belief systems about the functioning of my body, low self-esteem, as well as severe muscle tension from suppressing my emotional response.

The cumulative effect of all these traumas had a destructive impact on the energy systems of my body. Sessions with a healing therapist revealed that my basic energy grid—the foundational, structural energy pattern that surrounds the body—had ruptured. In addition, my field was torn in several places, including the surgical site of repeated diagnostic laparoscopies for infertility. My physical, emotional, mental, and spiritual bodies were no longer one, and due to all the damage in my systems, energy could not be contained in my field.

My energy field was defensively pulled upward and above my head, and the bottom edge of my field had shifted out through my back, behind my physical body. My lower five chakras were blocked, some disfigured, and there was no energy flowing through my pelvis, belly or legs. Energy flow through my meridians was disturbed, most notably the Gallbladder pathway. It is little wonder that I had suffered from arthritis, cancer, chronic fatigue syndrome, infertility, and depression.

With each traumatic event, more and more aspects of our energy become disrupted. When the grid is weakened, further trauma can be difficult to recover from. In particular, severe trauma or neglect that occurs in childhood can create significant disruption, as if creating a blockage between layers above and below, leaving a person feeling disconnected and isolated. However, while there can be qualities to these "layers" that are chronological in nature, there is no linear order.

In quantum physics, the study of the interaction of particles with light led to the discovery that these photons have both wave-like and particle-like properties, a paradox known as "wave-particle duality." Together, these seemingly contradictory properties provide a more complete understanding of particles. If we take into consideration this fundamental dual nature of particles—along with the quantum tenets that time is not linear and all possibilities exist simultaneously—we can understand how these "layers" of immobilized energy can have both chronological and nonlinear properties, regardless of the timetable of their initial creation.

Healing these layers of energy blockage is about allowing the body-mind to express whatever it is ready to, in its natural timetable, guided by innate inner wisdom. Of the body's healing wisdom, energy medicine teacher Roger Gilchrist writes, "It knows what it is doing from the time we are conceived until the time consciousness leaves the body."

Indeed, it is this "inner intelligence" that guides the healing process. As a healing therapist, it is not necessary for me to determine which layer to work with first. My role is to follow the process, and most importantly stay out of the way and allow healing to take place.

In an atmosphere of unconditional acceptance, layers of

blockages automatically present for healing, and healing energy automatically goes to wherever those blockages are.

We have seen how trauma can disrupt and even damage energy systems, and how the beliefs that result from trauma can disrupt energy flow. Now let's take a look at how trauma impacts our core, and why that is significant.

The Impact of Trauma on Core Energy Systems

As we have learned, our energy systems are organized around a central axis, which governs the formation of our physical and subtle bodies. Traumatic experiences can disturb this natural orientation to midline, creating measurable energy field distortion and disrupting the flow of energy through our systems. We know this has happened when we become oriented to the trauma or its aftermath, which shapes our identity and our beliefs. It is through our energy systems that we relate to the outside world, but trauma can cause us to bypass our own core, disrupting how we relate to our environment and the people in it. When we base our self-concepts on what others think of us and how they react and respond to us, we are not aligned with our core—our true source of power. When others become the source, the lifeline, or the "false God," we become dependent on them for approval because we are not "plugged into" our spiritual source through the chakra and nadis system. I sense these false lifelines as energetic "cords" that siphon away energy from our core.

In time, the innate orientation of our physical and subtle bodies to the core axis can be lost and a state of disrupted energy is accepted as normal. Our compensatory actions in movement and function also become accepted as normal. We begin defining ourselves in terms of trauma and thinking of ourselves in terms of limitations. This sense of limitation can become pervasive, coloring our view of the world. We can begin perceiving everything through the filter of limitations and scarcity.

When our identity becomes based on an energy blockage, rather than the truth of who we are as energy beings, health is compromised on every level. As our bodies become oriented to the energy disturbance, the flow of energy through the chakra and nadis system is disrupted, and we are no longer connected to consciousness or the flow of energy in the universal energy field. The result is tension, strain, and unbalanced movement patterns. When we aren't anchored in our core, we can be easily "triggered" by people and situations, knocking us off-center and disturbing our sense of balance. When we orient to trauma, a false identity forms based on being the victim of trauma. In essence, trauma can cause us to live a lie about who we are.

Brooke's story is an example of living a life based on trauma. Although craniosacral therapy had unwound the forceful impact of the car accident on Brooke's energy systems, relieving her dizziness and restoring the orientation of her field to midline, layers of earlier trauma still caused her to live an unbalanced life.

Brooke had few childhood memories, other than the sudden death of her mother when she was only eight, a trauma her father coped with through alcohol abuse. Forgoing marriage and children of her own, Brooke sacrificed her life to care for her younger siblings and her father full-time until his death. Brooke readily admitted she blocked out the past. "Why would I want to remember? It's not important," she said.

Brooke had been suffering from autoimmune disease, fibromyalgia, anxiety, insomnia, compulsive over-eating, and depression ever since her accident. It was clear to me that Brooke's unresolved childhood trauma had weakened her energy systems, making her vulnerable to the illnesses and diseases that developed after her car accident.

Despite the severity of her symptoms, all of Brooke's time went to others because doing otherwise and risking rejection and disapproval was unthinkable, even terrifying. Childhood trauma had resulted in Brooke's dependence on the approval of others. This dependency ruled every aspect of her life. Every decision she made in her personal and professional lives involved anticipating the reaction of others in order to prevent disapproval. Although she was only paid for an eight-hour workday, Brooke would stay after work and come in on her days off to prevent disapproval from her manager—even though he did not ask her to do these things. Between extending her work hours and changing personal plans based on the opinions and requests of friends and family, Brooke had no time or energy for self-care and any free time she had was spent in bed, exhausted and in pain.

When I looked at Brooke's energy systems, I understood her fears. Her dependency on the people in her life as her only source of energy was clearly visible to me as a cord that extended from the base of her misshapen solar plexus chakra—the energy center related to personal power—to those to whom she had handed over power and control. Brooke's sense of power through her core self, the power that comes from being connected to source, had been diverted to the people in her life. Her energy centers were closed, and she appeared disconnected from the universal energy field. (see figure 8-1)

No wonder Brooke was afraid of the disapproval of others. As she had become reliant on her family, friends, and work supervisor as her only source of energy, their disapproval was *starving* her energetically, as seen in her small and contracted field. She responded to this "energy starvation" by over-feeding herself with food. The excess weight that resulted from the overeating also served to protect Brooke from the deep hurt she felt from the disapproval of others.

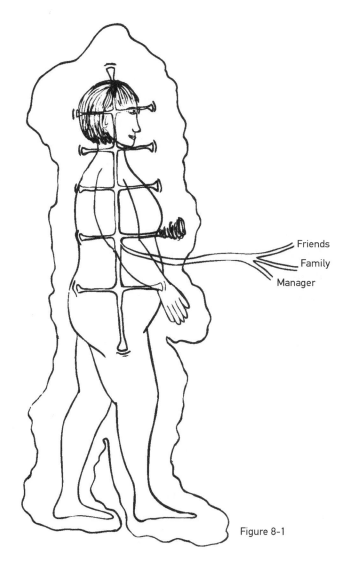

Friends
Family
Manager

Figure 8-1

While connection to the people in our lives through our energy centers is vital to our well-being, receiving energy from others is temporary nourishment at best, and draining, starving, or controlling at worst. Others can provide us with universal source energy through their own connection to source—such as during an appointment with a healing therapist or from our parents during childhood—but eventually we have to establish our own connection directly to source. As an analogy, if your car battery has "died," you become dependent on others to restart your battery through the connection of jumper cables to their car battery. But that is a short-term fix until your car can re-establish its own source of energy. It is through our connection to the universal energy field that we experience an *unlimited* source of energy.

In our work together, Brooke had an "aha" moment when she experienced a sudden, sharp headache at the exact same time that we discussed her compulsive need for approval. With that awareness, she spontaneously pulled her energy back from the solar plexus cord and into her chakra and nadis system, re-aligned with her core self, and re-established her connection to the universal energy field—right before my eyes. I observed Brooke plug into source through her crown chakra and to the Earth through her root chakra. All her energy centers opened with the restoration of energy flow through her core, and her field expanded out into the room. The experience of witnessing Brooke's dramatic unfolding was no less moving than witnessing an actual birth. (see figure 8-2)

Another issue associated with core energy flow disruption is known in holistic circles as *adrenal fatigue*. Symptoms of adrenal fatigue include fatigue, menstrual irregularities, mental fogginess,

temperature intolerance, food cravings, anxiety, and sleep disturbances. Although there are supplements effective at relieving such
symptoms, ultimately it is a disorder with energetic origins.

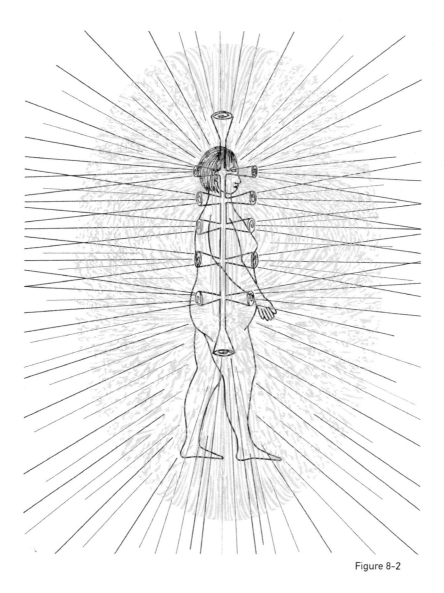

Figure 8-2

When core energy flow is disrupted from compromised energy systems, we tend to recruit adrenaline as an alternative energy source. However, the burst of energy produced by the adrenal glands is meant to provide us with *temporary* energy for a fight or flight response. When adrenaline becomes a *primary* source of energy, eventually the adrenal glands can no longer keep up with the demands for production. I liken this "burnout" state to a box of matches that cannot be lit because the abrasive strip on the side of the box used to strike and ignite the matches has been completely worn down.

Whether or not adrenal fatigue is recognized as a legitimate diagnosis in Western medicine is beside the point—compromised core energy flow compromises health. We cannot maintain adrenaline as a primary energy source any more than we can rely on friends, family, or managers to be our primary source of energy. Regardless of whether we have been energetically "starved" or are "burning" ourselves out, spiritual oneness with the universal energy field through our core energy flow is the solution.

Now that we've explored how energy blockages are formed—through trauma, beliefs, and suppression—and how these blockages can form layers and disrupt core energetic processes, it's time to examine the *healing* of our energy blockages—the process of shifting from suppression to acceptance that happens when we observe ourselves with compassion.

Even though I may have been taught to suppress my emotions, my body, my sexuality, and my negativity, and the impulse

to continue doing so is strong, I love and accept myself. Although this may be a lifelong pattern, I know it is energy-driven, and energy patterns are always changeable.

Even though I may be reluctant to express my emotions out of fear of appearing weak or fear of hurting others, I can always safely and respectfully acknowledge my emotions and fears with love and acceptance.

Even though past trauma may have created restrictions in my energy that caused me to view the world through the lens of lack and limitations, I lovingly claim my power to create and manifest abundantly in the world.

PART THREE:

HEALING ESSENTIALS

How Energy Medicine Can Heal You in Body, Mind, and Spirit

"All human suffering stems from the difference
between who a person says they are and
who they really are. This difference creates
a tension that functions like a black hole,
drawing in resonant people, places, events,
circumstances and situations in an attempt
to resolve the tension …we are all being asked
to transform ourselves to a new higher order
of increased harmony with the whole,
by resolving the difference between our actual
and potential selves."

—DON ESTES

~ 9 ~

ENERGY HEALING

"The body is a self-healing organism,
so it's really about clearing things out of the way
so the body can heal itself."

—BARBARA BRENNAN, PH.D.

"Then you will know the truth,
and the truth will set you free."

—JOHN 8:32

WE HAVE NOW REACHED the point in our journey where we can focus on the healing of disturbances in energy systems. The first eight chapters of this book have been like climbing a mountain, and we have arrived at the summit. Armed with the knowledge of the how, where, and whys of energy blockages, the view from the top is clear.

As we've seen, the impact of trauma can leave us with toxic, limiting beliefs. These negative beliefs create resistance, suppression, and non-acceptance, all of which disrupt and block the flow of energy. Clearly the path to healing and health lies in compassion, self-acceptance, and forgiveness.

The Steps to Health and Healing

To aid in the exploration of how we heal, I have translated the process into steps. Healing the disturbances in our energy involves:

first, awareness;

second, self-acceptance through compassion;

third, trust; and

fourth, surrender, a state of non-attachment that is a path to enlightenment.

As you will see, each of these "steps" becomes the pathway to the next.

By becoming aware of the signs of an energy block, and how we are being self-critical and self-rejecting, we have an opportunity to choose a different response—self-compassion and self-acceptance. In turn, self-acceptance creates trust, and trust creates a state of surrender.

It is important to note that this sequence of healing occurs *naturally*. The only action required to initiate the process is to choose self-love and self-acceptance. Once that choice has been made, being in a state of self-compassion instinctively instills a sense of trust and safety, and that sense of trust spontaneously leads to surrender.

Admittedly, choosing self-acceptance may not be that simple or easy, at least not in the beginning. Many people experience a strong initial resistance to accepting themselves. Nonetheless, we'll begin by exploring the four steps in the healing process one at a time, and later put them together holistically.

Awareness

As you've read this book, perhaps you've become more aware of signs that your energy is disrupted. To review briefly: Any physical, emotional, mental, or spiritual distress can be an indication of a disturbance in energy. This would include physical discomfort such as pain, tightness, and tension; emotional discomfort, such as sadness, fear, anger, guilt, shame, frustration, and feeling overwhelmed; mental discomfort in the form of negative thoughts; and spiritual distress experienced as a sense of aloneness or disconnection.

Whether or not an energy disturbance is transient or static depends on how we react to the distress the disturbance creates. If the distress is judged, criticized, and suppressed, the energy disruption will remain until trust is gained and acceptance can occur. If the distress is viewed with compassion and allowed to express, the energy disturbance is transient.

The Sword of Judgment

Whitney came to me near the end of her third pregnancy feeling run-down after four months of bronchitis that had not responded to repeated courses of antibiotics. I suspected the source of her blocked lung meridian and consequent bronchitis was grief, even though she did not appear sad. It took careful questioning in an atmosphere of unconditional acceptance for Whitney to admit how very sad she was.

When an ultrasound four months earlier had revealed her baby was a girl, Whitney had felt deeply disappointed. She already had two daughters and this had been her last opportunity to have a son. Whitney judged her disappointment as "wrong" and suffered tremendous guilt out of concern for how her response might affect her unborn child. Her belief that disappointment over her unborn child's gender was unacceptable was validated by close family members who sharply criticized her emotional reaction. To make peace, Whitney suppressed and silenced her disappointment, never speaking of it again. Four months later, she was unaware of the connection between the bronchitis she couldn't shake, and her suppressed grief.

When we suppress instead of accepting, we are unable to recover from trauma. Whitney was unable to heal from the traumatizing ultrasound findings because she did not accept her feelings. But how could Whitney begin the process of healing if she was unable to make the connection between her suppressed grief and her bronchitis?

Connections happen when we are in an open state. To complicate matters, the blocked-energy condition itself can block awareness. The solution isn't forcing us to become aware. In some situations, pushing ourselves to regain a frightening memory from an incident that is causing an energy disturbance can actually create additional trauma. Forcing is neither respectful of self nor compassionate, and does not build trust—and lack of trust *reinforces* an energy-disrupted state. In the same vein, allowing ourselves to stagnate in unawareness in order to avoid the discomfort that can accompany awareness is not respectful or loving of self either.

The question remains, how do you begin the process of healing *if you have no awareness of what is causing your distress*?

Insights can occur through gentle self-questioning, such as: What does this distress remind me of? When have I experienced similar feelings? What thought or belief triggered this distress? But tracing distress back to its trauma origins isn't actually required for healing. All that is required to initiate the healing process is to allow the distress you are currently feeling to fully *express*.

Allowing yourself to *feel* whatever you are feeling without judgment or criticism activates the healing process because emotions connect us with the energy disturbance that is creating the current distress. And within the energy wave pattern is all the information that governs the distress, the holographic nature of energetic frequencies, whether we are conscious of it or not.

When clients have judged and condemned themselves as "bad" or "wrong," and resist accepting themselves, I liken it to a house with all the doors and windows locked, the shades pulled, and the electricity shut off. There's no sunlight, no flow of air, and no flow of power. In this analogy, the house represents the energy field, the doors and windows symbolize the energy centers of the body, or chakras, and the electrical wires represent the energy channels, or meridians. If this state of resistance continues, the "house" can become moldy and filled with cobwebs and dust, and the air inside becomes stagnant. And since all possible entries are locked, no one can get inside to improve the condition of the house.

When a client is in a state of resistance, my job is to find an opening—somewhere, *anywhere*—in order to assist them. Since our physical, emotional, mental, and spiritual selves are interconnected, focusing on distressing symptoms on any of those levels can provide access. Even if the problem is primarily emotional, if the client is only aware of physical discomfort, that represents an unlocked window.

So even though the door to Whitney's grief was "locked," her awareness of physical discomfort represented an unlocked window, providing access to healing. And feeling compassion for the physical discomfort opens that window. Allowing the expression of discomfort—regardless of whether that discomfort is physical, emotional, mental, or spiritual—in an atmosphere of unconditional acceptance *initiates* healing, and that healing occurs on *every level*.

So we see that healing is about moving *toward* what causes us distress, even though avoidance may be our inclination. After a lifetime of effort to hold down, suppress, and control, it may not make sense to go *toward* distress, to let yourself really *feel* it or to even allow it to get *bigger*. But embracing distress with compassion is, in fact, the path to healing.

The Truth of the Matter

As you read about Whitney, you may have noticed your own beliefs about her situation. Do you believe, for example, that it's wrong to be disappointed about the gender of an unborn child?

When it comes to emotions, it's not a question of objective standards of right or wrong, it's a question of personal beliefs. So the question is always, "What is *my* truth?" You don't have to use any qualifiers or add conditions to justify how you feel. Simply put, whatever you believe is *your truth*. And it's important to be clear about your truth because what you believe forms the deep ground of your spiritual being, your core. And when we live outside of our center or core, or live weakly related to it, we create havoc within the energy system that is our body. When we become identified with untruths, this inauthenticity disrupts our essential orientation to the core axis within us, distorting the natural shape of our energy field and the flow of energy through our energy systems. To be inauthentic is to be out of alignment, or off-balance.

Revisiting the flowering plant analogy once more, it is our "flower" that opens in the vibration of personal truth and authenticity. Our flower closes in response to the energy of resistance. Taking it a step further, our "flower" cannot be "pollinated" by the metaphorical "bee" if it is closed in resistance. Manifesting, being "fertile," or "pollinating" in the world happens in the vibration of truth, where solutions miraculously unfold like the opening of a flower and we are fully engaged with life.

Both Whitney's concerns about the effects of her disappointment on her unborn child, as well as the disappointment itself, were valid. But in denying her true and authentic feelings, Whitney's baby was being gestated within blocked energy systems, by a mother sick with bronchitis.

From numerous documented accounts of individuals under hypnosis, we know that adults have the ability to recall vivid and emotional memories prior to their birth. The unborn do read energy and sense the emotional states of their mother. Certified hypnotherapist and professional counselor Michael Gabriel has "regressed" thousands of individuals who have had vivid and emotional pre-birth memories. As "proof" of their validity, in his book *Voices From The Womb,* Gabriel offers recorded pre-birth memories obtained through regression—information that was later verified by medical records and family members. In these situations, there was no possibility of the regressed individual having prior knowledge of the verifying information.

The question remains, how do you attend to your own need to express emotion while protecting an unborn child at the same time? In *Voices From The Womb,* Michael Gabriel writes, "What is the best advice I can offer you when you are pregnant? ...I would say that the best gift you can give your infant is to LOVE YOURSELF." On a more practical level, Gabriel recommends pregnant women communicate with their unborn child through a visualization process. By imagining yourself speaking to your child's spirit, you can build a relationship through communication of your feelings and experiences. But most importantly, the unborn need to know that whatever negative emotions or distressing situations their mother may be experiencing are *not* their fault.

When we tell a lie, the resulting disturbance in energy creates changes in our breathing, heart rate, blood pressure, and skin conductivity that can be read by lie detector devices. The energy disruption created by telling a lie also causes muscle weakness that can be perceived through muscle testing, or applied kinesiology, which we will discuss in chapter 14. This energy disturbance produced by inauthenticity is incompatible with health. For Whitney, denying her grief was, in effect, telling a "lie."

To demonstrate how "lying" creates an energy disruption, I'd like you to try this exercise. First, take an inventory of your body, noting how tense or relaxed you are. Now take a deep breath. On a scale of one to ten—ten being the deepest possible unrestricted breath—how would you rate the depth and ease of your breath? Write down that number. Now make an indisputably true statement, either out loud or to yourself, declaring your love for a person or a pet in your life that you love deeply and completely, without reservation...and notice how *that* feels. Picture this person or animal in your mind, and think about how much you love them. Now take a deep breath. Are you able to get closer to a ten? Do you feel less tense and more relaxed?

Now turn your statement of love around and make it false by stating that you don't love them at all. As thoughts are energy, just the thought of stating this lie may be enough for you to experience the disturbance in your energy. Take another deep breath as you think or repeat this lie. Has your number rating for depth and ease decreased? If you continue to think or say this lie, you may notice a sense of weakness, tension, or even a twinge of pain. You have just created a transient energy disturbance. If you return to thoughts of love, it will be gone as quickly as it came, but you can imagine the toll of suppressing your authentic feelings every day.

All told, a lack of self-acceptance effectively closes the door to healing when energy flow is disrupted. And suppressing our emotions as a result of this non-acceptance locks that door. Not accepting ourselves disrupts the flow of energy through our energy systems, disturbs the natural orientation to the core axis, and creates a disconnection from the universal energy field. But accepting ourselves restores energy flow, opening the door to healing.

The Role of Compassion

Accepting the truth of who you are and what you are feeling creates an opening for healing to occur, but knowing the importance of self-acceptance for your health and well-being does not necessarily get you there. When you realize you aren't accepting yourself, your first impulse may be to criticize yourself for not accepting yourself, which creates more non-acceptance!

When we ask, "Why can't I just get over this?" we are judging ourselves. Love the part that's having difficulty "getting over" your issues, as well as the self-critical part that is judging you for having the issue.

When you pay close attention to your inner dialogue, you may find that you are constantly finding fault with yourself and others. When you judge yourself like a critical inner parent, the child within can't trust, and trust is necessary for surrender.

Now I want to clarify here what I mean by "judging." We constantly judge ourselves and those around us as a means of classifying, interpreting, and gaining a sense of control in our lives. The problem comes when we judge and then *condemn*.

The pervasive issue of judgment in our culture has its roots in Judeo-Christianity, upon which Western society is founded. In the last one hundred years, an "emerging paradigm" of Christianity has viewed a relationship with an unconditionally loving God as the path to transformation. But for many Christians, their beliefs come from what biblical scholar Marcus Borg refers to as the "earlier paradigm"—a view of God as "Lawgiver and Judge" whose acceptance has conditions. In *The Heart of Christianity*, Borg writes, "We most often put conditions on God's grace: God accepts you *if* . . . And whenever an 'if' clause is added, grace becomes conditional and ceases to be grace." Likewise, when we put conditions on loving ourselves and others, it *ceases* to be love.

When we consider this belief in a judging God, we can see how such a weighty paradigm would influence the deep-spirit level of our being, and how we perceive and treat ourselves and others. What results is self-judgment—often harsh judgment—and that will most definitely affect our energy systems, often in a way that seriously compromises our health.

If you feel blocked and are judging and criticizing yourself for your feelings and behavior, please know there is *always* a valid, underlying reason why we do the things we do, and why we feel the way we feel. Judging and criticizing our feelings and behaviors dramatically disrupts energy flow. It's that simple and that dangerous. To give you an analogy, judging yourself with condemnation is like throwing a car into reverse while you are driving. Not only does it stop the car dead in its tracks, it does serious damage to the vehicle.

Judging and criticizing keeps our fears hidden and suppressed, and disowned and projected onto others. Both responses block energy flow. Accepting and loving creates inner trust, which allows the hidden fear to surface where it can be expressed, accepted, and then released. But before the hidden fears can surface, our deeper selves must trust that we won't be judged and condemned. Gaining that trust involves developing habits of self-acceptance.

The path to self-acceptance lies in *compassion*, including being compassionate with the part of you that is resisting acceptance, and compassion for your distressing symptoms. To observe with compassion is to witness without conditions, expectations, attachments, or resistance. As we know from quantum physics, this is an act of creation. Observing yourself is like *watching* a movie versus *being in* the movie. When we are *in* the movie, we are living a story about ourselves, and we lose objectivity. When we are watching the movie, we are in the position of the *higher* self, versus the *lower* or "ego" self. In the higher self, we have objectivity, we are aware, and we see the bigger picture.

In Whitney's story, initiating healing began with feeling compassion for her physical symptoms, her irritated lungs and the restrictions in her breathing, as she was unaware of her suppressed grief. At first, Whitney expressed hatred for her lungs. I see this frequently in my work, clients who feel their bodies have "let them down." The offending body part then becomes the enemy. Have you ever felt angry for stubbing your toe? Or referred to a body part as "stupid" because it's not working "right," or to your expectations? As we know, all emotional responses are valid and meant to move through the body with the flow of energy. However, when we direct anger or hatred at our body parts, we isolate those parts from the flow of energy. As long as you see your body as your enemy, you cannot heal.

Once Whitney realized that what her inflamed lungs needed was *compassion*, not hatred, her energy began to flow and she was able to express her underlying grief, which brought her to the second step—acceptance.

Awareness of her physical distress represented an unlocked "window" in Whitney's "house." In feeling compassion for that physical distress, Whitney was able to let go of resistance and suppression, which opened that window. And as light and air could begin to flow through the window, they provided access to turn on the "electricity," the flow of Whitney's energy, and begin the process of unlocking more doors and windows in her "house," restoring health and vibrancy to her body-mind.

Compassion as the Bridge to Acceptance

"I hate being fat," said Sophie. "Why would I accept that I'm overweight? That doesn't make any sense. I want to lose weight, not stay fat."

I can certainly understand how Sophie would feel this way. After all, I was once in her shoes, and adamantly resisted accepting my excess weight. So when I talk about acceptance, I am not talking about excusing or condoning the behavior of overeating. The behavior is not the primary issue. Let me explain, using an example.

Withholding acceptance because we believe that accepting ourselves as we are will perpetuate a situation is the same as not responding to a baby's cries to prevent it from crying more. As we have learned, the cries of an infant are an attachment-seeking, acceptance-seeking, or love-seeking behavior. There was a powerful reason why Sophie was overweight. Her overeating behavior came from deeper-level emotional wounds, which cry out for love and acceptance. This is the level at which acceptance must come in. By accepting the part of you that is hurting or frightened and soothes itself with food—that uses excess weight as protection—you gain access to healing those parts.

Claire was harshly judging and critical of herself, as her parents had been. Her frequent infections, fatigue, and insomnia, as well as her difficulty in expressing herself verbally, had all contributed to Claire's tendency to hold herself back, which made her feel hopeless about accomplishing her goals. Claire was unable to ask for a raise at work, unable to go back to school to further her career, and even unable to adopt a dog, which her children had been requesting for two years. From time to time, Claire had convinced herself that getting a dog would be a good idea, but she had not been able to take any action in that regard.

As Claire talked about her frustration while lying on my healing table with my hands laid on her, I began to discern a fear vibration in Claire, which I sensed was coming from a young part of her. I asked Claire if we could dialogue with the child within her.

"Do you see 'Little Claire'?" I asked.

"She's hiding."

"Where is she hiding?"

"She's in her bedroom. The door is closed, and she's cowering on the floor behind the bed."

"Knock on the door and see if she would be willing to talk to you."

"She's afraid."

"What is she afraid of?"

"She's afraid I'm going to judge her."

"What do you think she needs to hear?"

"I think she needs to hear that I won't judge her."

"What is her response to your reassurance?"

"OK, she's let me in."

"What does she need to trust you?"

"She says she's still afraid I'm going to judge her."

"Ask her if she can give you a sign when you are judging her, so you can self-correct."

"She says she will pull on my arm. She says—*watch for a twinge in your arm.*"

I want to note here that working with the "inner child" can be controversial. Psychologists and counselors know that people can get stuck psychically when early trauma occurs and they become identified with the wounds of the child. There is a school of thought that "killing off" the inner child is the path to healing. However, I have found that healing the inner child happens through compassion and acceptance from the higher self, which creates *integration.*

Acceptance Creates Trust

Immediately after completing this exercise, Claire had a spontaneous memory of bringing home a stray dog when she was about seven years old. The dog had a skin infection which it passed to her brother. Rather than treat the infection, Claire's mother had the dog euthanized, and forced her to watch, telling her it was her fault that the dog was going to die. The situation was so traumatic that Claire had unconsciously repressed the memory ever since.

We had established trust by dialoguing with the frightened part of Claire, and in response that part of her offered up a memory that had been buried for decades. She could either judge and criticize this memory, or have compassion for it. By showing compassion, she built trust within herself.

By the end of the session, Claire's resistance had released, and she felt eager to take action toward her goals. The next time I saw her, Claire had happily adopted a dog, to the delight of her children. With that breakthrough, the pattern of holding herself back in life began to dissolve. After a few false starts, she enrolled in a university, started playing the piano again, and found her voice by singing in a church choir.

To my senses, judging with criticism creates a spiral of negativity that locks down our energy in layers. Judgment tends to beget *more judgment*. I liken this spiral of negativity to twisting a length of fabric until it is compressed and hard. The way to undo this compressed spiral until it unfolds and softens is to love every part of yourself, even the part that is critical and the part that feels criticized, until there is nothing left out of the love equation.

Claire shared with me her own analogy for healing self-judgment:

"It's like if you stand between two mirrors, you will see an infinite number of selves in your reflection. When I'm judging myself, and then judging myself for doing so, it can seem like a never-ending cycle of judgment, like I'm between two mirrors that reflect judgment over and over."

"Yes, that's right. And by looking in that mirror with love and acceptance, that love can create a never-ending cycle of acceptance that heals," I added. When we apply the high energetic frequency state of love and acceptance to the low energetic frequency states of shame, guilt, apathy, grief, fear, desire, anger, and pride—we raise our energetic frequency level to the realm of health and happiness.

Trust Creates Surrender

I would like to give you another example of how trust leads to healing.

A year after becoming a first-time dog owner, I felt ready to help another shelter dog. But the calm, friendly, and well-behaved dog we adopted didn't seem to need my help. At first, Stanley appeared fine. But his calm exterior was deceiving.

Stanley began pacing in front of doors and windows, and rapidly losing weight no matter how much he was fed. Beagles tend to be overweight due to their preoccupation with smells and food, but Stanley was one skinny beagle.

Puzzled by his behavior, I noticed that although Stanley craved human companionship, he did not accept anyone's affection for more than a brief moment, and showed no preference for the company of us over strangers. When I touched him, I noted that his muscles were hard and tense and he didn't seem comfortable in his body or with his surroundings. And along with the pacing behavior, Stanley began compulsively gulping water from his bowl and wanting to go outside to relieve himself, sometimes every fifteen minutes.

After weeks in this energy-disrupted state, Stanley's health began to deteriorate. He developed recurrent eye infections and a bout of inflammation in his neck that caused severe pain and necessitated emergency intervention. The veterinarian could find nothing medically wrong that would account for all his strange symptoms. What was happening to my dog?

It took time for me to recognize that Stanley had a canine version of attachment trauma and was failing to thrive. Stanley was no different than the babies studied in Romanian orphanages who withered away for lack of love, or the children with attachment trauma who display "indiscriminate affectionateness," characterized by an excessive familiarity with strangers.

We only had information from the most recent seven months

of Stanley's life, and the number of living situations he experienced during that time could certainly have accounted for his attachment trauma. Earlier in the year that we adopted him, Stanley had been removed from a high-kill animal shelter by a rescue group. He was placed in the rescue group's private shelter, then adopted, only to be returned to the shelter within four months, and then finally adopted by us. I suspected that after experiencing repeated separations from people he may have bonded to, Stanley had begun to protect himself by avoiding attachment. But how could I help a dog heal from attachment trauma?

Even though in my daily work with clients I seek to establish trust as part of the healing process, I didn't initially recognize that the same was needed for my dog. In order for Stanley to attach to his new family he had to trust first, which would require more focused action on my part. Now I'm no expert in dog behavior, but the way I saw it, in order to gain Stanley's trust, I needed to show him what I wanted him to do—attach to me.

To help Stanley, I asked him to stay close to me by keeping him on a short leash at my side. Holding the leash created both a physical attachment between us, and kept him physically close to me. He struggled for half an hour, pulling at the leash to get away and avoid closeness. This is the same struggle I see my clients go through, that struggle to let go that precedes release. Throughout the time that Stanley struggled with the exercise, I stayed relaxed, patient, and completely accepting of him, allowing his resistance to fully express as needed. When he finally let go of resistance, Stanley flopped down on his side, close to my body, and let out a deep sigh. He had surrendered.

As I rewarded Stanley with a massage, I could feel his muscles relax and observed the tension melting from his body. For the first time since we adopted him, Stanley closed his eyes and rolled on to his back, exposing his belly in a sign of trust. As I witnessed this moment of healing, I was moved to tears. Stanley could finally take in the love I offered.

I repeated the short leash exercise several times over the following few days, each time asking him to stay close to me for a while. With my intention and through my actions, I asked him to trust me. Each time Stanley surrendered more quickly, just as my clients are more quickly able to reach a state of release with experience.

Stanley's compulsive pacing, drinking and urinating stopped, his painful neck condition and chronic eye infections resolved, he regained the lost weight, and he began to seek me out on his own for more sustained close contact. But best of all, Stanley became the relaxed, healthy, and happy dog he was born to be, securely attached to us and his dog sister Lexi.

As Cesar Milan, *The Dog Whisperer,* says, "You never get the dog you want. You get the dog you *need.*" Stanley fulfilled a need I didn't even know I had—a need to understand the healing of attachment trauma on a deeper level. I believe he came to me not only to receive help for himself, but also so I could help others, through the sharing of his story.

As we saw with both Claire and Stanley, once trust was created, surrender occurred *spontaneously.* But for many of my clients, the concept of surrendering, or "letting go," is foreign.

The Meaning of Surrender

When I talk about surrendering with a client, the responses I frequently hear are, "I can't surrender, because...

- I'll lose control."

- I'll go crazy."
- I can't just stop meeting my responsibilities and obligations."
- I'll lose my passion."

As you may recall from chapter 3, Steven was afraid of losing his mind if he let go. This is a common fear I encounter in my work. Others are afraid that if they surrender, they will lose their passion because they have mistaken resistance and fighting for passion.

Sometimes, beneath the fear of letting go are the fear of the unknown and the fear of death. Indeed, surrender has been referred to as "the little death." When we surrender, we drop into our center and experience oneness with the universal energy field, a preview of the oneness awaiting us with the death of our physical bodies. When we are in resistance, we are removed from that experience of oneness.

In previous chapters we met Helen, who didn't feel comfortable talking about her feelings. She believed that in order to stay positive, she had to resist her sadness. Helen was attempting to stay in control by holding it all together, but doing so only put up a wall around her emotional self. "What do you mean surrender?" she asked. "I can't just stop managing my father's care. I can't just give up on doing my job. I have to stay on top of everything, including all the infertility appointments and medication schedule."

Helen resisted my attempts to work with her energy blockages, and remained very tense throughout the session, leaving my office with layers of suppressed energy flow. She could not allow herself to be vulnerable because she did not trust in the process of healing.

Although I didn't feel like I had helped Helen, I believe healing always happens in the right time and in the right way.

The next time I saw her, I was surprised to find most of Helen's energy blockages had released. All her chakras were spinning, her field was expanded and oriented to the core axis, and her energy was flowing. She was more relaxed than I had ever seen her and was practically beaming. "Has anything significant happened since the last time you were here?" I asked.

Helen described a recent cancer scare that proved to be unfounded. "It put everything in perspective," she said, "and I just feel so grateful for my health and everything in my life." A month later, Helen called with news that she had conceived through previously unsuccessful allopathic infertility treatment.

How did Helen heal? Although she hadn't felt comfortable exploring her feelings about her infertility or past sexual trauma in our work together, her willingness to consider another way of viewing her situation had created an *opening*, in effect unlocking one of the windows in her "house." When faced with the possibility of a life-threatening health issue, her focus had shifted fully to the present moment and the traumas in her past had lost their hold on her. In this way, the health scare had served as a catalyst for healing. Without even trying, she had let go of the past and let go of resistance.

When we are tied up in trauma from the past, we function in survival mode. Helen's energy had been bound up in resisting her emotional response from past trauma. When she let go of the past, resistance was released and her energy became available for the present moment, the energy required for growth and creation. So we see that surrendering means letting go of *resistance*, not letting go of your obligations, responsibilities, or passions. To let go of resistance there need only be a willingness to consider situations in a new light.

All body processes function optimally under conditions of surrender. This is best illustrated when considering functions around reproduction. Mammals will cease reproducing if they are under severe stress and don't feel safe. The labor process will also halt in mammals who feel they are in danger. This response to danger is also seen in humans.

Many bodily processes require a state of surrender to function optimally, such as sleep, childbirth labor, the sexual response, and the milk ejection reflex in breastfeeding. It is only when we are in a state of disrupted energy flow that results from resistance that these natural bodily reflexes are blocked. As such, surrender is a natural state. Anything else is resisting "what is." Even "trying" to achieve this natural state of surrender is a form of controlling.

It is through letting go of control, including trying, that surrender occurs.

And in finally surrendering to *"what is,"* we flourish.

Even though I may have judged, minimized, trivialized, or criticized and suppressed my emotions in the past, I now choose to restore energy flow by treating myself with kindness, gentleness, patience, and compassion.

Even though I may have difficulty accepting myself as I am, I can begin the self-acceptance process by focusing on what I consider my positive attributes. That focus of acceptance connects me with the Divine, and through that connection I become the source of change.

Even though I may be afraid of losing control, losing my mind, losing my passion, or losing my life if I surrender, I can build the trust within myself to do so by compassionately and unconditionally sending love and acceptance to my fears.

～ 10 ～

HEALING THE VICTIM

HOW LOVE, RE-PARENTING, AND
RADICAL FORGIVENESS HEAL

"In all my years of inner and professional exploration,
I have come to know that compassion for yourself is the key to
true happiness, and not feeling it is the source of much depression,
anxiety, addiction, and low self-esteem."

—KATHLEEN HANAGAN, L.C.S.W.

MY FIRST BOOK will never be published. It was a memoir that chronicled the traumas of my life in great detail, including the sixteen-year struggle with infertility. After completing the manuscript, I sent it to an editor for review. Although the analysis I received deemed the book well-written, there was also criticism, the harshest of which was directed at the main character—who of course was me. In the manuscript I had come across as a victim, and an angry, domineering drama queen.

At first I responded in true victim fashion—feeling attacked, criticized and rejected. But at the same time that I was upset over the evaluation, deep down I knew she was right. Although the book contained a powerful message of healing, the bulk of the story was so steeped in victim consciousness it wouldn't have been helpful to anyone. I could see how those who felt victimized would have identified with my story—but rather than being uplifted, I feared the book would only have served to keep them in that victim place. The wounded little child part of me had taken over the writing project from the first word. It had become a vehicle for her voice, and she had a lot of say.

I loved my first book. I loved every carefully chosen word. It was precious and perfect in all its imperfections. I had worked with it with the same tenderness one would show a baby. And I grieved the decision not to publish as if I had lost a baby. The purpose of sharing my story was to inspire and help others, but I had completely missed the mark.

During daily walks through my neighborhood, my tear-filled eyes hidden behind sunglasses, I tried to make sense of what had happened. My chest hurt at the thought of two years' wasted time and effort, all that I'd poured into the book in the name of helping others, all for *nothing*.

As I pondered this, a small voice within said, *"Aren't you worth all that time and effort?"*

Startled, I almost stopped in my tracks, but continued at a slower pace as I considered this message. Could it be that the countless hours I had invested in writing what I thought was for others was actually an investment in... *me*? Was I really *worth* that much work and effort? In an instant, I knew the answer: Yes, I am.

I began to recognize this pattern of feeling criticized and rejected by authority figures in my life; from my parents, nursing school instructors, work supervisors, and many others—most recently the manuscript evaluator. Each of these individuals had been mirroring my belief that I was unworthy of acceptance, through what I perceived as criticism and rejection. What they were mirroring back to me was the small, angry self who had suppressed her anger for years. Decades. And now that angry, hurt self had unleashed her rage and hurt through the pages of the book.

No wonder the poor editor had been put off by my "voice." For sure, it had been the voice of *The Victim*.

But now... now a new perspective had dawned. I *was* worth *someone's* time and effort—my own. And fortified with the awareness that I *was* worth spending time on, I decided to revisit my now-defunct writing effort, and look at it a little more objectively. So I asked myself, *If I'm worth investing time and energy in, what did this investment in me give... just to me?*

Thinking about it, I began to see how writing a book that no one would ever read was, in fact, the *perfect* medium for fully expressing the victim story. I got to vent; no one had to be subjected to it. And the critical evaluation?—that was the *perfect* means for helping me let go of that story. Moreover, I saw how I had experienced the behavior of all these authority figures throughout my life through this "frequency of unworthiness" that vibrated strongly in my energy systems. Any authority figures I had been in contact with who matched my vibration in unworthiness received my projection and mirrored it back to me. And in the same vein, I recognized that I had unwittingly been the receiver of others' projections of unworthiness, mirroring it back to them through *my* rejection.

Finishing my walk that day, I marveled. By revisiting the rejection of the manuscript in a new frame of mind, I had been given an opportunity to heal, not only from the trauma of failed effort, but also to deepen the healing from many prior traumas. I felt a sense of gratitude for the experience and all that I had gained from it, and in that moment I realized forgiveness for the events of a long, difficult past had occurred.

Healing "The Victim"

Now when I talk about forgiveness, I don't mean forgiveness in the traditional sense. What I mean is *radical forgiveness*, a term coined by Colin Tipping, author of a book of the same name and founder of The Institute for Radical Forgiveness Therapy and Coaching.

Traditional forgiveness comes with the assumption that someone has done something wrong and needs to be excused or pardoned. In *radical forgiveness*, there is no obligation to forgive, no sense of righteousness, no pretense, no denial, and no requirement to condone the offending behavior or situation. Rather, forgiveness happens through insight, when we see situations for what they are—opportunities for growth.

According to Tipping, "True forgiveness must include completely letting go of victim consciousness." Once I fully expressed the grief of the "death" of my first book, I realized there was nothing to forgive, because nothing was "wrong." I had received a gift, the gift of transcending the victim.

Not only did the book's failure serve to expose and heal victim consciousness, it also opened the way to a profound experience of self-acceptance. When I could see the editor's evaluation of my character as only a reflection of one thing—*my own sense of unworthiness*—her criticism no longer mattered. It wasn't a criticism of me as a human being; it was a statement about a voice that had come out of me. I realized that every part of me was valuable and worthy of acceptance, even the part that is prone to bouts of anger, the part that is drawn to drama, and the part that longed to have the whole world validate her victimization. In loving all the "me's" in the book, I learned to truly love every part of myself.

In accepting all the parts of myself represented in my memoir, I realized that even referring to these aspects of me as "parts" was only an illusion, because there is no separation. And by giving a voice to and being accepting of all the wounded aspects of myself, I no longer needed a public forum to air my pain. When we embrace every aspect of ourselves with unconditional love— we heal. As self-judgment and criticism create fragmentation and *disintegration*, self-acceptance and love create wholeness and *integration*.

Spiritual Connections

All the authority figures throughout my life who I had felt rejected by were serving as my spiritual partners. Indeed, we are all connected through the medium of the universal energy field, and assisting each other through spiritual connections, even when that "assistance" creates trauma. When others unconsciously accept our projections, sometimes at great expense to themselves, they help us grow. In this way, trauma can become the *vehicle* for healing and transformation, and by healing the victim, we heal *trauma*.

Revisiting the *Big Bang Theory*, if every particle in the universe was once compressed into a tiny ball, then even though everything is now spread out over the entire universe, we remain interconnected; we remain one. As such, you are a part of everyone, and everyone is a part of you. When we identify ourselves as victims, and others as perpetrators, we remove ourselves from this oneness; we create disturbances in our energy systems. Similarly, when we identify aspects of ourselves or parts of our bodies as the enemy and feel hatred toward that part, we remove that part from the oneness and create major disruption in our energy systems.

The truth is, even when we distance ourselves from others through victim consciousness, we are never actually separate. But when the flow of energy is obstructed through victim mentality, it does create the feeling of being cut off and separate. This is the illusion of separatism. Healing this sense of separation occurs through *compassion.*

A young teen with learning disabilities I worked with had suffered recent trauma from a physical attack by an older boy who taunted him with the insult, "You're weak." The younger boy responded as a victim—feeling angry, hurt and powerless.

"Why would he hurt me? I didn't do anything to him!" the boy said. I suggested that his attacker may have been responding to a vibration of "weakness" in the young teen, as the bully may have felt weak himself.

"He may have been bullied too, although that's no excuse for what he did. Maybe he was trying to prove his strength by attacking you," I continued. The young boy recalled once punching a friend in the arm to prove his own strength, in response to being called weak.

"The way to vibrate in strength is to imagine yourself as strong, and feel what it would be like to be strong, not to prove your strength by hurting others," I explained.

As he pondered these ideas in the context of his own experiences, the young man began to feel compassion for his attacker.

A few weeks later, something amazing began to unfold. In a letter of apology, the bully wrote that he knew how his victim must have felt because he had also been the victim of bullying. As the victim put himself in his bully's shoes, the bully was now putting himself in the victim's shoes. The boys then formed a "friendship club," and sealed their bond through a handshake ritual. Through compassion, their relationship transformed from victim-victimizer to partners.

Ultimately, healing trauma is about healing victim consciousness, which happens when we realize there is nothing to forgive. But let's back it up a bit. Forgiveness has to come freely. We can't just blanket over resentment, which is another form of suppression. We have to fully express ourselves first, through the meeting of unmet needs.

In the previous chapter the healing process was broken down and presented as sequential steps for ease of explanation. As such, these four steps of healing that lead to true forgiveness are *awareness, acceptance, trust,* and *surrender.* These are not linear steps, however. In this chapter these aspects of the process of healing will be considered as a whole, taking the information to a deeper level.

Parenting Ourselves

We have explored awareness in terms of becoming aware of disturbances in our energy systems. In order to heal these energy blockages that result from trauma, we need a deeper level of awareness—an awareness of our unmet needs. To heal these disturbances, we need to give ourselves what we didn't get. Why? Because as long as our need for love, acceptance, security, safety and trust remain unmet, our development can be arrested. And

being in a state of searching to meet those needs outside of ourselves disturbs our essential orientation to our core selves.

When we grow up, we take over the job of parenting ourselves,
based on our perceptions of how we were parented. To recognize
your unmet needs, it is helpful to look at those perceptions. If you
perceived your parents as rejecting, rigid, inconsistent, or not sensitive to your needs, then healing begins with becoming aware of
how you may be rejecting, rigid, inconsistent, or insensitive with
yourself—and then fulfilling your need for acceptance, flexibility,
consistency and sensitivity. Making the choice to become sensitive
to your own needs *includes* consistently accepting the parts of you
that are rejecting and rigid.

In other words, if you felt rejected as a child, then healing is
about becoming aware of how you may be rejecting yourself, and
making a choice to accept yourself unconditionally. If you feel
you were treated rigidly as a child, then healing is about becoming
aware of how you may be rigid with yourself, accepting that, and
making a choice to treat yourself with flexibility. If you feel you
were treated with inconsistency as a child, then healing is about
becoming aware of how you may be inconsistent with yourself,
and making a choice to become someone you can rely upon and
trust. And if you felt insecurely attached to your childhood care-
takers, then healing is about creating security within yourself.

The truth is *no* parent can 100 percent meet their child's
needs. It's not humanly possible. As such, healing is accomplished
through *re-parenting* ourselves with compassion, through our
spiritual connection. Meeting our needs then becomes an inside
job, and in meeting those needs, we build trust and a sense of
security. If past trauma has left you feeling devalued, unaccepted,
unloved, unsafe, insecure, or untrusting, then healing is about

valuing, accepting, and loving yourself, which creates a sense of security, safety and trust.

The Effects of Unmet Needs

It is important to work toward fulfilling our own needs, because as long as we continue looking outside ourselves to fulfill our needs, we will never get there. Why? Because vibrating in the frequency of "unmet needs" attracts more "unmet needs"— through people and situations that contain a match for that vibration. When we fully accept ourselves as we are, we fulfill our unmet need for love and acceptance. In doing so, our energetic frequencies begin to vibrate in fulfillment, attracting people and situations that match that vibration.

But if you never received unconditional love, how can you give yourself unconditional love? If you were raised with rejection, how do you stop the cycle of self-rejection? This is the challenge of the healing process.

Using the flowering plant analogy I have used for energy systems, when you are traumatized in childhood, it is as if your "plant" is not fully developed. How do you meet your own needs if your energy systems are like drooping leaves on an underdeveloped stem with withered roots and no flower? How can you connect with the universal source of energy in such a state? The answer is through *compassion.*

Fulfillment

When we can have compassion for ourselves and others, we release the victim and gain access to healing, personal power, and spiritual growth. It is through compassion that we connect to the universal energy field. Through compassion our life force is activated. Through compassion our underdeveloped "roots" and "stem," or base chakra and central nadi, can indeed flourish; our "leaves," or energy centers, can unfurl, and our "flower," or crown chakra, can bloom. With compassion we can let go of our ego attachments and the false "lifelines" that drain our energy, and restore flow through the core, reconnecting to source. Through compassion, kundalini energy flows, energy centers open, the energy field expands, connections happen, and we experience *oneness*.

Although compassion is the key to fulfilling unmet needs and healing, it's not always easy to get there. However, looking at how secure people respond to stress can be helpful.

When securely attached individuals feel angst, they conjure up images of the parent to relieve stress. In this regard, thinking about someone who gave you a sense of security works just as well, whether that is a person living or passed, or a spiritual connection to a deity. Many of my clients who were insecurely attached to their parents had a more secure attachment to their grandparents or other extended family members or family friends. Imagining that person in times of distress can create a sense of support. For others who lack a secure attachment to someone they knew personally, that feeling can come through imagining a spiritual icon, or through nature experiences, where they most strongly feel a spiritual connection. But ultimately, fulfilling our needs is about learning to treat ourselves in a way that does fulfill those needs. Let's take a look at some examples of fulfilling unmet needs.

Sophie put unflattering pictures of herself on her fridge, in an attempt to motivate herself to stick to her eating and exercise plan after gastric bypass surgery.

"How do those pictures make you feel?" I asked.

"It makes me feel bad. It makes me hate my body."

"Who would you feel more motivated to work hard for—a boss who makes you feel bad about yourself? Or a boss who is kind, compassionate, and supportive?"

"A boss who is compassionate."

"Do you think it is effective to motivate yourself by putting pictures on your fridge that make you feel bad?"

"I see your point," said Sophie.

As Sophie and I worked together to correct the disturbances in her energy systems, she became more aware of her body and emotions. She learned how to sense the energy disruptions created when she treated herself harshly. Hating her body created a sense of tension and heaviness, while self-compassion created a sense of lightness, peace, and happiness.

Sophie began to realize that in hating her body she had created a block to the very thing she desired—a thinner body. When she resisted the reality of her excess weight, energy flow was disrupted. In time, Sophie learned a new way of being with herself. Each time she noticed critical thoughts about her body shape and size, she asked herself—what wounded part of me is this critical thought coming from? And what does that wounded part of me need in order to heal? The answer was always the same....*love*.

The Shadow Self

Healing the victim also involves becoming aware of what we have disowned, what we consider our "darkness"—what is hidden in the "shadow."

As I am not a psychologist, I want to point out that my use

of psychological terms like "shadow," "projection," and "narcissism" may be slightly different from how a professional in that field might use them, and are not meant to be diagnostic or to quantify pathology. Rather, I use these designations to facilitate understanding of energy dynamics in the context of healing, as I have come to understand them as an energy medicine therapist.

It is important to heal our shadow selves, because if we continue to live with this split inside of us created by disowning parts of ourselves, we are living a major underlying energetic imbalance that can result in poor physical, emotional, mental, and spiritual health.

Health is about achieving balance through embracing both the dark and the light within us. This harmony is depicted in the Eastern yin-yang symbol, in which light and dark teardrop-shaped halves each contain a smaller circle of the opposite color. Enlightenment is about taking ownership for what we believe and for our behavior, dealing with the consequences, and accepting ourselves as we are. In this way, we bring that which is in the shadow to light and achieve healthy, mature personhood. Energetically, enlightenment activates the flow of energy through the nadis and chakra system and connects us to the universal energy field.

Discovering our shadow material is by no means an easy process. Although doing so may require professional assistance, we can discover what is hidden by looking at our dreams, which we will discuss in chapter 14, and through becoming aware of what we are *projecting* on others. By observing ourselves and how we react to certain people or situations, we can obtain clues about our shadow material. As such, the questions to ask yourself are: Is this situation upsetting me because of something I can't accept in myself? Does it remind me of a past traumatic experience? Am I feeling jealous of someone because they are doing what I wish I could do, but am afraid to? Or does this interaction help me realize that a part of me is underdeveloped and unexpressed?

Once we become aware of what we are projecting on others, the shadow self has been exposed. The next step in healing the victim is taking back these projections and claiming them as our own, with compassion and acceptance. When we make the choice to stop blaming others for our current situation, and take responsibility for what is ours, the victim is healed. Disowning and hiding disturbs energy flow. Bringing the hidden parts of ourselves into the light creates energy movement.

The Shadow Story

When we disown and suppress our authentic selves into the shadow, we unconsciously create a "story" about who we are. Living this story causes energy disruptions and blockages that disturb our orientation to core—creating a "disorientation" about who we are and a sense of disconnection from the universal energy field.

Regardless of the traumas we have experienced in our lives, there remains a part that is untouched. This is your core, the essence of who you are, located in the physical and energetic core of your body. When we are aligned with this core, our energy systems are open and connected to the universal energy field. But when we are living a shadow story, we are not oriented to this core. Becoming reoriented is about letting go of the stories we have made up about ourselves. In letting go of the story, taking back our projections, and bringing what is hidden into the light, we heal.

We think that in order to be loved and accepted we have to become someone we are not. But the truth is—sharing our authentic self actually makes us more "attractive." When we are aligned with who we really are, our energy systems vibrate harmoniously, creating a magnetic attraction.

Mandy attended a highly competitive high school. To gain acceptance and compensate for feelings of inadequacy related to her family's past bankruptcy, she began pushing herself harder and harder in school. Praise from her parents, peers, and educators propelled her forward to reach greater and greater heights—higher grades, more awards, and faster times on the swim team—even though attaining those accomplishments meant getting only a few hours of sleep a night, and living a miserable, unhappy, and empty existence. But Mandy could not stop her pursuit of achievements. They had become her identity, a story that defined who she was.

What followed in Mandy's life were a series of traumatic disappointments. Despite all her hard work, she was not accepted at her top choices for college, nor was she offered a scholarship. At the college where she was accepted, Mandy continued her pattern of seeking achievement, but her grades were disappointing. She turned her focus to getting into a sorority, only to be further disappointed when she was not accepted by any of her choices. She had worked so hard to achieve acceptance, but all her efforts seemed to be failing. What had happened?

Mandy was no longer able to gain acceptance through achievement because her efforts were based on the illusion that the path to love and acceptance was through becoming someone she was not. With each new disappointment, the illusion that she had staked her identity on began to collapse. Mandy plunged into despair and hopelessness, and felt utterly alone—the experience of the dark night of the soul, a stage that can occur in the process of healing.

In time Mandy emerged from the dark night, only to be confused about her identity. Without her achievements, who was she? This is the transition stage of the healing process when the old has ended but the new hasn't yet begun. As she explored her authentic self, gradually old beliefs were replaced with new ones. She realized that what she desired in life bore little resemblance to what her peers desired. Achievements and material acquisition were no longer a priority. Her focus had shifted to how she could best use her talents and education to serve humanity.

By letting go of resistance and surrendering, Mandy realized she had nothing to be disappointed about, as everything had happened in the right time and the right way. She knew that neither her top choices for college nor joining a sorority would have been right for her. She was indeed in the perfect place. What she had interpreted as disappointments were actually experiences she had unconsciously attracted as part of her healing process. These experiences were ultimately for her highest good. In time Mandy began to rebuild her life based on authenticity.

Mandy's story shows us that healing the shadow is about the *acceptance* of both what is in the light and what is in the dark.

Revisiting Acceptance

As we have learned, self-acceptance is a vital step in healing. All parts of us exist as a part of the harmonious whole, and *we* exist as part of the greater harmonious whole. However, when we do not accept every part of us, there are consequences. Nature provides us an illustration of this concept, specifically an herbal plant. When scientists isolate the "valuable" active component of a complex plant from the inactive components to create a medicinal drug, a substance that was once part of a healing herb can be potentially deadly, as it lacks the natural system of checks and balances inherent in the whole plant.

In nature, every part of a plant is valuable, and every species in an ecosystem is valuable. We are also a part of nature and, as such, every part of us is valuable. When a part of a plant is isolated from the whole, when a species is eliminated from an ecosystem, when a part of us is repressed and hidden in the dark—we upset the natural order and disturb the health of the whole.

We are like a tapestry of many different woven threads. If you look closely at the threads, you may find some you don't like. But if you start picking apart the threads you find unacceptable, the tapestry will begin to unravel. When viewed as a whole, we see how all the different colored threads of the tapestry work together to form something beautiful and balanced. Accepting every part of us is like appreciating the rich tapestry of who we are. But for some, unconditionally accepting and loving ourselves sounds too much like narcissism.

Self-love Versus Narcissism

"Why is self-love so important?" asked Sophie. "Being in love with yourself doesn't sound so great to me. I can't stand people who are so conceited they have to constantly tell everyone how beautiful and amazing they are. I never want to be like that."

I can certainly understand Sophie's confusion about self-love. When someone truly loves themselves, they are secure in that knowledge and have no need for excessive admiration from others. Such love of self is based on unconditional acceptance of one's authentic self, not based on accomplishments or physical appearance.

As we heal, there may be times that we need to be overly self-focused in order to attend to our unmet needs. This would be considered *healthy* narcissism, when a self-focused individual continues to show concern for others and has goals in life. This is different from *pathological* narcissism, in which that self-focus interferes with life goals and can cause indifference toward others than can range from selfishness to outright exploitation.

However, it is important to note that for those who have been traumatized, feeling compassion for others can be an issue. When so much of our energy is directed toward fulfilling our own unmet needs for love and acceptance, it can leave little energy for others. Developing compassion in and of itself then becomes the route to healing. On the subject of cultivating compassion, Buddhist monk and former cell biologist Matthieu Ricard says, "An analogy is the pure love that a mother has for an innocent child. You let that grow in your mind, so there's an all-pervading compassion. At some point, non-referential compassion becomes a state that you can generate in your mind."

And so we see that it is through awareness, acceptance, trust, and surrender that victim consciousness is healed. And in healing the victim, we heal trauma, thereby creating the health and happiness that results from authenticity.

You will know you have begun to heal the victim when you experience the feeling of gratitude, an element of forgiveness. However, as healing is an ongoing process, there will always be more layers to heal, and more opportunities to accomplish this healing. In the next chapter, we will examine important characteristics of this ongoing process.

Even though I may have blamed myself, others, or God for the difficulties in my life, I recognize this blaming game as victim consciousness and know there is nothing to forgive.

Even though I may be reluctant to love myself out of fear of narcissism and self-centeredness, I accept myself and understand that self-focus may be necessary in my process of healing.

Even though I may have been attached to struggle, control, or perfectionism and these attachments may have become my identity, I love and accept myself just as I am. I am beginning to recognize my attachments as an illusion and a false identity, and trust in this process of becoming who I really am.

~ 11 ~

THE HEALING PROCESS

"Healing is a process. It is about rocking back and forth
between the abuse of the past and the fullness of the present
and being in the present more and more of the time."

— GENEEN ROTH

THROUGHOUT THIS BOOK, I've noted that healing is a *process.* This idea can be difficult to understand in the West, where healing is commonly defined as the removal of a physical, emotional, or mental symptom—an *eliminative* process. All too often we circumvent real healing through popping pills, or through practices that emphasize positive thinking over dealing with our wounds.

As such, there is inadequate information in our culture about healing as a *transformative* process. This dearth of information is far-reaching, having existed for nearly four generations, since the publication of the Flexner report. Given this, aspects of this process can seem foreign, and even peculiar, to Westerners. This can create difficulties in recognizing when healing is actually occurring.

As a professional with years of experience working in the healthcare field, I once believed that healing meant symptom elimination. It wasn't until I experienced this process for myself and studied it in a naturopathy program that I grasped healing as a continual process of clearing, releasing, integrating, and growing—a *way of life*. In this chapter, I would like to begin to share with you some of the important aspects of this process that I have discovered. As such, the healing process is:

- Ongoing
- Multi-level
- Dynamic
- Unexpected
- Inside-out

Within these categories are other characteristics and patterns. Let's begin with the *ongoing* nature of healing.

Ongoing

Healing is not a destination, not a point to reach. To help illustrate this concept, I will use the Illness/Wellness Continuum developed by John Travis, M.D., a pioneer in the wellness movement.* Imagine a continuum, a line extending infinitely in both directions, with a neutral point at the center that symbolizes the absence of discernible symptoms of illness. Achieving this neutral point of "non-sickness" is the goal of allopathic medicine. However, staying at any point on the continuum, including the neutral point, is actually stagnation.

---

*His continuum model can be found in *The Wellness Workbook: How to Achieve Enduring Health and Vitality,* which he co-wrote with Regina Sara Ryan, a wellness writer and former nun.

Further, the point you currently occupy on the continuum is less significant than the direction in which you are facing. The important question to ask is this: Are you moving in the direction of illness and premature death, or are you moving toward awareness and growth? You can be symptom-free, yet progressing toward illness; or disabled, but in the process of healing. You can live a great life with your condition or be limited by it. I've come to see a whole range of healing, from a completely transformed life free of symptoms on every level, to growth and awareness in the midst of disability.

Vanessa was raised by emotionally neglectful parents. Her healing from such severe and prolonged emotional deprivation throughout her childhood has been long and difficult. She frequently expresses concern over how much longer it will take for her to be "done." But when Vanessa focuses on healing as an endpoint, she shifts from being in the flow of her healing process to being in a state of resistance.

I lost sight of my own process during my experience with infertility. I became so focused on achieving my goal of pregnancy that I put my life on hold. Living in this state of limbo while waiting to be "done" created stagnation and my personal growth slowed to a snail's pace.

I didn't realize: Life *is* the process.

Deidra was so debilitated by chronic fatigue and fibromyalgia that she had been unable to work outside the home. Although Deidra is in the process of healing the many blockages in her energy systems related to childhood sexual abuse, she still has bouts of fatigue and pain. Even so, her life has changed dramatically since beginning her healing process. She no longer expends all her energy on the caretaking of others, but has found balance in her life through self-care. Deidra has achieved high coherence with the universal energy field, and experiences that singularity as synchronicities in her daily life.

When Deidra visits the library, she thinks, "*What can I find here today to help me on my path?*" Then she "lets go" of any pressure or expectation of finding anything—yet is inevitably drawn to a particular book that speaks directly to whatever issue she is currently dealing with. Even though Deidra still has bouts of pain and tension, she is highly aware of her body and how situations trigger her. She is compassionate and accepting of herself, and in a state of non-resistance. Deidra is on a journey of self-discovery and healing.

Earlier in this book, we looked at the dynamics of healing within a client session. But the process of healing doesn't necessarily *begin* with a session—nor does it take place exclusively *during* a session. The process begins with the first intention of healing—when we seek answers to our physical, emotional, mental, and spiritual issues—and continues through self-care practices and professional healing therapy.

What's important to note is this: Whether or not that process continues unabated depends on how well-established it is. Depending on the modality of the healing therapy, the skill level of a practitioner, the nature of the energy disturbances, and the commitment level of the client to making changes, a single session can be enough to activate inner healing resources and establish a continuous healing process. But usually it takes multiple sessions, especially when there are many layers of energy disturbances present. In that situation, the client may notice marked improvement in their issues for a few hours to a few days, and then lose ground due to the influence of remaining energy disturbances.

But with each appointment, the length of time spent in a state of improvement increases.

The pace of healing is largely determined by the level of acceptance. Clients who lack self-compassion and are resistant to accepting themselves and their situation remain in a state of blocked energy until they are able to begin accepting themselves, whether that takes days, weeks, months, or years. If you already have self-empathy, healing will progress more quickly. But if you don't, it can take time to develop, and self-empathy doesn't happen by judging yourself for not having it. It begins by focusing on something you do like about yourself. Are you a caring friend? A compassionate parent? Talented at a hobby? Passionate about a cause? Excel at your career? When you focus on what you consider your positive characteristics—that represents a window that can be opened; a window into healing.

When the process is well-established, healing can continue indefinitely, unless further trauma takes place. This pattern of improvement is usually gradual, but once it gains momentum, there may be instances of healing that can be quite dramatic. In this dramatic healing, significant improvement can happen almost instantaneously.

Later in this chapter and the next, I will relate the story of my son Jacob's healing, and the quantum leap in healing he experienced when he was about six years old. We will also look at some healing principles from naturopathy and homeopathy, illustrated through the story of my healing and Jacob's. But first, let's look at other aspects of the healing process.

Let me add something here in reference to how men approach the healing process. By and large—they *don't* see it as a process. Maybe it is because of the more mechanical way many men tend to approach the world (added to the fact that men generally do not like to discuss emotions), but many males want healing to be a quick, measurable event. "How many sessions will this take?" is a common question that therapists of all disciplines hear from their male clients during the first visit.

I must reassure all readers, healing is a process. One, or two, or three sessions are not likely to resolve life or energy issues that took years to form. Healing is a way of life involving mindful awareness coupled with healthy physical, emotional, mental, and spiritual choices, and incorporating natural self-care practices for energetic vitality.

Multi-Level

As we have seen, blockages in energy systems affect all levels—physical, emotional, mental, and spiritual. Likewise, when we heal, that healing occurs on every level, as healing is by its very nature *holistic*. In essence, there is no such thing as "physical healing" or "emotional healing," because there is no separation between our physical, emotional, mental, and spiritual selves. All our "parts" are interconnected, and we are interconnected with all of life.

"I must have hurt my back at work," Jim said on the phone. "I think I need to cancel my appointment so I can stay in bed and rest," he added. Because the focus of previous sessions had been on emotional issues, Jim assumed I only worked with emotional pain. Once I explained that I work with any type of pain, he kept his appointment.

During Jim's session, at the moment I asked him about his emotional state, his back pain suddenly and dramatically increased. The connection between his emotional angst and physical pain was unmistakable to both of us. There is no difference between emotional pain, physical pain, mental pain, or spiritual pain. Pain and illness have the same origin—disrupted energy flow.

While working with Tess and her arthritis, inflammation, unexpressed anger, and critical tendencies, she related her struggle with hateful thoughts. At the same moment that she spoke of these hateful thoughts, the area of her body where she had just had a wart removed began to throb. According to Louise Hay, teacher, lecturer, and founder of Hay House publishing, warts are about "little expressions of hate." Her book, *Heal Your Body A-Z: The Mental Causes for Physical Illness and The Way to Overcome Them,* contains a thorough index of physical conditions and the mental beliefs that cause them. Once Tess found compassion for her hateful thoughts and allowed herself to express them, the pain disappeared.

If your only sign of healing is the cessation of a physical symptom, then healing has probably not taken place. Either you aren't aware of the other signs of healing, or the symptom was only suppressed, leaving the root cause unaddressed. In true healing, there is involvement of all levels, as we shall see in the stories throughout this chapter and the next.

Dynamic

As healing is not a point to achieve on a continuum, neither is it a set point on a *scale*. Health is a naturally dynamic state that *includes* the experience of illness. If you were to chart how you feel throughout each day—physically, emotionally, mentally, and spiritually—using a scale of plus five to minus five; you would notice that over time, the ups and downs balance each other out. Our natural state is to seek equilibrium.

It is not natural to be consistently up, consistently down, or to have wide swings in mood as seen in bipolar disorder. For those who feel generally flat, or mostly hyper, their healing can emerge as an expression of this natural balancing pattern. This change can initially feel strange, and even frightening.

As she began healing, Vanessa noticed that her sense of well-being varied throughout the course of her day. After a lifetime of feeling emotionally flat, she thought there was something wrong with her. For the first time in her life, she was experiencing natural fluctuations in her mental, emotional, and physical energy levels. For others this pattern of ups and downs may have always been present, but they were unaware of it until they began healing.

In nature, this pattern of perfect balancing is called the *meandering pattern*. This law of nature is found in such varied forms as a winding stream with its equal number of left and right turns, the pattern of lightning, and the arrangement of cranial sutures (joints between the bones of the skull). In the movement of water, this pattern slows down the flow for the support of life and is associated with the filtering and oxygenation of water. Water that flows too quickly creates erosion; water that flows too slowly creates stagnation. And just as surely as a meandering stream shapes the landscape, so to do the cycles of our lives shape our inner landscape.

Ancient cultures created labyrinths, a type of maze that features the meandering pattern. Walking a labyrinth helps us align with the natural equalizing rhythm within us, creating balance.

Another pattern I have noted within the meandering pattern is the pattern of *rising baseline*. You might have noticed this pattern at work in the process of healing from an injury or from surgery. Although recovery from these events naturally follows the meandering pattern of ups and downs, the baseline of well-being will steadily improve until full recovery is achieved unless healing is obstructed. This can create a sense of "one step back for every two steps forward."

With certain drugs, particularly anti-inflammatory medications, healing from injury or surgery can lack the full expression of the natural meandering pattern. While it may seem advantageous to eliminate the "downs" and only have "ups," the variability aspect of the meandering pattern is vital to health. In fact, measurements of physiological variability are reliable indicators of state of health. For example, in *Tapping the Healer Within Us,* Roger Callahan, Ph.D. writes, "Cardiological research has determined that the greater the variability in the heart rate, the healthier the heart, and the more stable and healthy the body."

For those actively engaged in a healing way of life, the pattern of rising baseline is applicable in a much broader context. Let's revisit our imaginary scale for a moment, in which we rated how we are feeling throughout each day from plus five to minus five. Given that the meandering pattern represents perfect balancing, you might assume that the baseline of this scale, or the "zero" point, would remain fixed in our lives. Indeed, there are many scientific studies that indicate just that. These studies show that the baseline of one's "happiness scale" is set for each person, and does not change over their lifetime. Whether you get married, have a baby, or win the lottery, you eventually return to your previous level of happiness, as if we have a "set point." However, these studies were conducted on average *Westerners,* not on individuals engaged in the process of healing as a way of life, nor on those experienced with meditation.

Although happiness research is in its infancy, it is clear that the positive life events and material acquisition that we usually associate with happiness only create temporary improvement in our moods. Lasting and increased happiness is associated with positive interactions and connections with others, especially when those connections are associated with acts of generosity and compassion. As you may recall, compassion is a vital aspect of the healing process; the bridge to self-acceptance. Compassion is the emotion that creates connection to others.

This association between compassion and happiness is born out in a study of Buddhist monks with years of experience in meditating on compassion. While engaged in this meditation, brain activity in an area of the left prefrontal cortex associated with happiness eclipsed activity in the area of the right prefrontal area associated with unhappiness. Changes in brain wave activity associated with heightened consciousness were seen even when the monks were not meditating, indicating an enduring change.

In my own experience, as well as those of a number of clients I have worked with over long periods of time, I have noted a change in the baseline of happiness. My level of happiness has steadily increased over the last twenty years, and continues to do so. Peak experiences of joy occur more frequently, and my set point continues to climb higher. What I rated as a "plus" experience on my scale twenty years ago is more like a "zero" on my scale today.

Unexpected

Healing often occurs in ways we couldn't even imagine. Instances of healing can happen any time—while reading a passage in a book, hearing a particular song on the radio, experiencing an act of kindness from a stranger, or during an encounter with nature. Time and again, clients report that issues resolve in ways they least expected. You may recall that quantum physicists have discovered that an infinite number of possibilities exist at once. We choose the possibility of healing with our thoughts and emotions by thinking and feeling as if we are already healed. However, in this process of creating our life, it is important to be in an accepting state, detached from the details of how and when that healing will occur. Why is this so?

If we decide in advance how and when healing is to take place, we are resisting all other possibilities for resolution, and it is this very state of resistance that disturbs energy flow. When we try to figure out how issues will be resolved or direct our healing, it is a form of control. And when we trust that an issue will miraculously resolve, even if we don't know how or when, we are in the process of healing.

My Experience

I would like to offer several examples of this unexpected nature of healing from my own life. It may help you see the surprising ways that the steps of healing can present in our lives.

For many years, I was stuck in a state of resisting my infertility. Since I equated letting go with giving up on completing our family, I refused to surrender to the reality of our situation.

Earlier, I related my experience of encountering "the wall," which felt like being trapped in a circular room—my perception of blockages in my energy systems. Each door in this room represented a possibility for resolving our struggle with family-building. Some of the doors took me nowhere, others were locked, and I resisted entering the doors that were unlocked. Unfortunately, determining my options in advance, represented by the doors, only served to maintain the disturbances in my energy. It kept me trapped in the circular room of my mind because, as it turns out, the series of three unexpected events that would lead to resolution weren't represented by any of the doors!

These events began to occur after engaging in intuitively guided rituals of grief work. Through this deep expression of grief, I began to develop trust in the idea that however our infertility journey concluded would be acceptable. I began to realize that no matter what happened I was going to be OK And with that trust, after years of resistance, I took my first tentative step into letting go.

The first occurrence began with clues that appeared in my dreams—recurrent nightmares that I was a serial killer. At first I was too horrified by these dreams to make sense of them. But when the nightmares persisted, I began to pay closer attention.

When I considered the content of the dream as a metaphor, I could see how the "killer" within me could be the system of the body that "kills" pathogens and tumor cells—my immune system. Could the dreams be telling me that my immune system was malfunctioning? Was my body repeatedly "killing" embryos developing in my body? To find out, I requested immunological testing through a holistic medical practice. The tests revealed the presence of anti-ovarian and anti-adrenal antibodies, indicating an autoimmune condition. But even more significant, my natural *killer* cell (NKC) count was highly elevated, a condition known to cause early pregnancy loss by inhibiting implantation and the early formation of the placenta.

The conventional medical treatment for an elevated NKC count was, and still is, intravenous infusions of immunoglobulin G, or IVIG, at a cost of thousands of dollars per infusion. IVIG temporarily suppresses the NKC count, necessitating repeat infusions about every four weeks. This treatment wasn't covered by our health insurance carrier. So although the message in the dreams had led to a diagnosis, there didn't appear to be an acceptable solution. Pondering this situation, I asked for another message to appear in my dreams to guide me.

That very night, a man approached me in a dream and said, *"Expect a miracle."* The dream was so vivid I awoke with a start in the pitch-dark. I had no idea what form that miracle would take, of course, but I knew it was coming.

The following day I related the lab results and my puzzling dreams to my acupuncturist, Amber Rose, Ph.D., L.Ac. She suggested I try apitherapy, or bee venom therapy, a treatment successful in facilitating healing in the immune systems of individuals with multiple sclerosis. Unbeknownst to me, Dr. Rose was a pioneer in combining bee venom therapy with acupuncture in the U.S. The use of live honeybees to treat acupoints instead of needles is documented in her book *Bee In Balance: A Guide to Healing With Honeybees, Acupuncture, and Common Sense.* "Bee-acupuncture" has been used by the Chinese for over 3,000 years. Apitherapy was also practiced by Hippocrates, considered the Father of Western Medicine.

Prior to this, if anyone had suggested I allow myself to be stung by live honeybees as a mode of healing, I would have told them they were crazy. I was terrified of bees. But there I was, in a state of non-resistance, going with it. Years later, this time in my life came up in conversation with a friend. She related how she was genuinely concerned for me and thought I had "gone off the deep end" when I mentioned I was using bee venom therapy as an infertility treatment.

Within four weeks of beginning bee venom therapy, my energy level increased dramatically and the chronic fatigue syndrome appeared to go in remission. Blood tests revealed anti-ovarian and anti-adrenal antibodies were no longer present, and the NKC count was within the normal range. While the suppressive effects of IVIG only last about four weeks, the healing effect obtained from bee venom therapy has been permanent. My immunological lab values have remained at a normal level ever since.

After the elevated NKC count had resolved and months went by without conception, I reached a deeper point of surrender. We had done everything we could, short of unaffordable IVF, and there was nothing left to try. I wasn't ready to give up, but I had no idea what else to do. In an act of letting go, I threw out all the infertility-related materials that I had accumulated over the years.

A few weeks later, a second event occurred that would bring the situation closer to resolution. A memo arrived in the mail, along with my paycheck, detailing changes in my health insurance coverage that would cover three cycles of IVF. This represented a totally unexpected turn of events.

There had been an "IVF door" in my mental circular room. However, the only possibilities that I had imagined for obtaining the "key" for that door were either moving to a state that mandated coverage for infertility or winning the lottery. Never had I imagined obtaining coverage through my current job. By deciding those were my only two options for proceeding with IVF treatment, I became bound to how our infertility was to resolve. In this attached state, I remained blocked for years, stuck in the circular room until I detached and let go of trying to control *the manner* in which resolution was to take place.

Tragically, the first two cycles of IVF failed to produce a

viable pregnancy. It would take everything I had learned to experience these traumatic losses in a way that did not block my energy systems. Although it is human nature to become attached to the outcome of these cycles, regular appointments with healing practitioners during these treatment cycles kept my energy open and flowing and in a state of detached non-resistance.

The day I received the news that the second cycle had also failed I allowed myself to fully feel and express the grief, without reservation. As I did, I reached a deep level of letting go. From the abyss of grief, I reached out with a prayer, asking for however Jacob was meant to come into our family to be revealed to me… no matter what it was. In that moment, for the first time since we had begun our infertility journey, perhaps for the first time in my life, *I was in a complete and total state of surrender.*

I was in that state when, suddenly, a surge of powerful and startling information from the universal energy field "downloaded into me"—and in an instant I knew how to alter our last IVF treatment cycle to create a body for Jacob's soul. Without identifying the source of my information, I delivered the different approach to my reproductive endocrinologist. And although he was surprised by my suggestions, he agreed to the change in strategy. I acted on the intuition that came through in that moment of surrender and, in doing so, Jacob was conceived in our third and final attempt at IVF. The miracle foretold in my dream had come true. The six-year journey to give my son life had at last concluded.

Learning this lesson of non-resistance is one of the many gifts received from my infertility experience that serves me well to this day.

Now I'm not suggesting that women with infertility and elevated NKC counts should use bee venom therapy. The point is to be open to the unexpected, and not rely solely on the specific treatment regimen you have chosen. It is through that openness that our answers are revealed, whatever they may be.

For me, being in a state of openness required trust—trust that was built over time. Healing the blockages in my energy systems opened the way for these events to occur by decreasing resistance. Letting go of resistance was an incremental process, until I made that quantum leap to surrender on the day I received the news of our second IVF failure.

As it happened, bee venom therapy also made it possible for me to have a complication-free pregnancy the third time around. Despite being told I had virtually a 100 percent chance of developing pre-eclampsia, an immune disorder of pregnancy, as I had developed it twice before, my immune system functioned normally.

Inside-Out

Jacob began to exhibit puzzling behavior within months of his birth. As an infant, he was unusually rigid and impatient in his feeding patterns, behavior that lactation consultant colleagues had never seen before in their practice and were at a loss to offer guidance.

After receiving his six-month vaccinations, Jacob's development seemed to stop. He lost the ability to babble, showed little interest in his toys or surroundings, cried for most of his waking hours, vomited frequently, and rarely smiled. The calendar I kept to record the developmental milestones of his first year of life, as I had done with my other children, was completely blank after that initial six months.

Not only was I concerned with Jacob's behavior and development, I grew increasingly alarmed with his misshapen head, cranial asymmetry also known as plagiocephaly. His head looked like taffy pulled diagonally with bulging on both the right side of his forehead and the back of his head on the left, and flattening of the back of his head on the right side. A serendipitous encounter in a local store with a former healing school classmate brought a referral for craniosacral therapy when Jacob was nine months old. Craniosacral therapy is the light touch therapy that works with the core structures of the physical and subtle body (discussed in chapters 4 and 5).

Jacob showed signs of improvement with his very first cra- niosacral therapy session. Prior to therapy, the pressure on his vagus nerve created by his asymmetrical skull bones had caused him to vomit up to twenty times a day and scream when placed on his stomach. Since he was unable to lie on his stomach, he was unable to learn how to crawl.

As Jacob was growing and gaining weight at an above average rate, (no doubt due to my overabundant milk supply, an unusual situation), his pediatrician was unconcerned about the vomiting, or perhaps doubted the frequency. His vomiting decreased to two to three times a day after the first craniosacral therapy session and stopped completely after the second session. Over time, as we continued therapy, his head became symmetrical.

I had the privilege of witnessing Jacob's release of birth trauma at nine months of age during one of his early craniosacral therapy sessions. While the therapist was gently working with the bone at the top of Jacob's skull, images of his birth flashed through my mind: the vacuum extractor attached to the top his head, the obstetrician pulling on the extractor to facilitate the birth of his ten-pound body, and the way Jacob looked completely spent when finally freed from my body. I saw the worried expressions of the nurses and obstetrician over his bluish color, his poor muscle tone, and his rapid, labored breathing.

At the same time those birth images were flashing through my mind, Jacob began to scream, his face bright red as he unleashed deep, angry wailing. I felt his rage pass through me as a wave of energy. I held him and wept as he released the trauma of his difficult birth.

Jacob's release experience exhausted him and he fell into a deep sleep in my arms, waking later with an expression of peace on his face, so different from the seriousness I had thought was his natural state.

While Jacob's issues initially presented as physical asymmetry in his skull and vomiting, they had impacted every area of his life. And as he healed, the changes were seen in every area. Not only did his development resume, with the return of verbal babbling and his learning to sit up and crawl, but his curiosity returned. He became engaged in his life; eager to learn, move, and explore.

Hering's First Law of Cure

With craniosacral therapy, Jacob had healed from the inside-out, consistent with the first tenant of Hering's Law of Cure which is considered to be the basis of all healing in homeopathy. This law of healing dictates that healing progresses from the internal to the external; or from deeper within the organism to the superficial parts. For example, depression that lifts and is followed by a skin issue is progressing according to this law of healing. In Jacob's case, the asymmetry that had been visible from the *outside* of his head was an expression of the imbalance and restrictions present *inside* his skull. Once that imbalance and restrictions were released on the inside through craniosacral therapy, normal function was restored, and the resulting change was reflected on the outside with a symmetrical head and improved function.

The allopathic treatment for "flat spots" of the skull involves the use of a molding helmet that applies pressure on some areas of the skull to encourage flatter areas to round. Helmets are worn up to 23 hours a day for six to 24 weeks. With this molding helmet treatment, change is directed from the outside-in. In natural health systems, this approach would be considered a *violation* of the first rule of Hering's Law of Cure.

When health issues are treated with suppression, whether molding helmets or suppressive drugs, the condition can be driven deeper into the body. When joint inflammation that has been treated with anti-inflammatory medication is followed by a heart valve issue, or an individual with eczema who is treated with suppressive medications later develops multiple sclerosis—both are thought to be examples of violations of the first rule of Hering's Law of Cure. As we have learned, when the body's natural healing progression is repeatedly suppressed, eventually it can no longer rally, and the condition can become chronic. In the naturopathic viewpoint, chronic conditions are seen as the direct result of suppressive treatment.

Spiritual Partners

After Jacob was born, I looked back with fresh perspective through the dream journals I had kept throughout my infertility struggles, recognizing themes for the first time. I noticed numerous entries regarding dreams of having twins. When Jacob was born, it was as if I was reborn with him—a twin birth of twin souls, Jacob and I. In the first years of his life, more aspects of our spiritual partnership would be revealed.

In the next chapter, we will look at those aspects as we explore more laws and principles of healing.

Even though I may have thought there is only one path to healing, I realize the possibilities for healing are limitless and I choose to embrace the path for growth that has presented in my life.

Even though I may be afraid of losing control, balance, or steadiness in my life if I allow patterns of variability to express, because being flat and even feels safe, I love and accept myself. I trust in the natural up and down rhythms of life and healing.

Even though I may have been trying to figure out and control how my issues will resolve, which inadvertently creates obstruction in my life, I love and accept myself. I trust that all will unfold in the right time and in the right way.

~ 12 ~

HEALING PRINCIPLES

"Every encounter provides you an opportunity to create authentic
power, but when your encounters include others who
are also using their experience to create authentic power,
the potential for spiritual partnerships comes into being."

— GARY ZUKAV

"WHY IS IT THAT I FEEL an instant attraction to one person and am repelled by another?" Vanessa asked during her energy healing session. "I mean I understand that I'm sensing energy, but then there are people I feel nothing toward at all when I meet them. Am I only sensing energy with certain people?"

To answer Vanessa's question, we need to delve further into this concept of spiritual connections and partnerships. You may think that a spiritual partnership is about a lasting love connection, but we experience spiritual connections with anyone who creates an impression—positively or negatively. Even if contact is only brief with someone who is otherwise a stranger to you, who you never see again, or if your reaction is to a public figure who you have never actually met—if you are "triggered" by another, energy dynamics are at work.

Just as how we *feel* gives us information about the state of our energy systems, how we *react* to others does as well. We are always sensing energy, whether our reactions are positive, negative, or neutral. Those whose energetic frequencies are a match for our positive or negative frequencies unconsciously mirror back to us whatever state we are vibrating in—whether it's unloved, unworthy, unvalued, unsafe, or unable to trust—or loved, worthy, valued, safe, and trusting. For those who aren't a match for our frequencies, the response is neutral.

The valuable information we glean from these positive or negative reactions that occur through our spiritual connections can assist us in our healing process—helping us discover our shadow selves, uncovering our hidden agendas, showing us where our issues or layers of issues remain, or validating where we are in our healing process. What is happening when we react negatively is touching into each other's garbage, or filtering through our "stuff." Moment to moment, we are either responding to others from a place of fear or a place of love.

It is when we become conscious of our spiritual connections and actively use them with others for mutual spiritual growth that we form the type of spiritual partnerships Gary Zukav describes in *Spiritual Partnership: The Journey to Authentic Power*. The conscious creation of authentic power through these cooperative partnerships is the highest expression of the healing process.

Spiritual Connections and the Healing Process

In this chapter we will be continuing our exploration of spiritual connections and partnerships, as well as the principles and ongoing nature of healing. As we continue our survey of Hering's Laws of Cures, these principles of healing will be illustrated through the story of Jacob's healing and mine with vibrational medicine.

From the beginning of my infertility journey, it seemed Jacob's spirit was assisting in my path to enlightenment, preparing me to be the mother he would need. It was a perfect partnership of him assisting in my healing, so I could in turn help him. Encouraged and amazed by his response to craniosacral therapy, I decided to become a craniosacral therapist myself. It was the core body therapy I had been searching for to complement my skills in working with the energy field and energy centers.

As I studied craniosacral therapy, I had a moment of super-objectivity where I seemed to grasp the greater picture of our lives. Flashes of insight came to me unbidden. I began to realize that Jacob had, in effect, been assisting in my education as a healing therapist from the very beginning, preparing me for my role in the world. It was through his difficulties that my eyes were opened to how powerful we all are, even a baby. The thought that my child would do such a thing for me literally brought me to my knees.

Giving him life was my main motivation to continue my healing process, no matter how difficult or how long it took. If he had arrived sooner, I would have lost my motivation to carry on with healing the disturbances in my energy systems, because I did not think myself worthy of such effort. I didn't think I mattered, and I put my children's needs ahead of my own. In time, I would begin to heal this frequency of unworthiness, but until then, the hope of bringing Jacob into this world served as motivation to stay engaged in my process. Indeed, our attachment to outcomes can keep us motivated to stay with our healing process, but ultimately there will come a point in our healing journeys when that attachment must be shed in order to continue.

Obviously, I had much more daily contact and personal connection with my own child than I would with a client. However, an energetic bond does form between healing practitioners and clients that is important to the healing process. Facilitating healing involves being energetically merged with a client in a spiritual partnership, while maintaining boundaries.

Layers of Issues

I had hoped that Jacob's healing was complete when the cranial asymmetry was healed, but I was beginning to understand that his plagiocephaly was only one layer of his issues. I was beginning to grasp that his healing was a process. But there was more to the story. Not only was I learning from Jacob how to be his parent, but from the very beginning of our long journey in family-building, I was being prepared for a calling I never would have dreamed of or chosen had I not walked this path.

Those were the intuitions to ponder. There was more healing to come in terms of letting go of personal negative beliefs that could interfere with parenting a high-need child. I was learning how to become more assertive, thanks to Jacob's condition. From the day he was born, I had to step out of my comfort zone and advocate for him with the newborn intensive care staff and physicians, our pediatricians, and the many other professionals who would become part of his recovery. In order to be effective, I had to begin to step out of the victim role.

Although Jacob's development resumed with craniosacral therapy, his development was slower than expected and he was well behind his peers. As he grew into a toddler, the rigid and impatient behavior I had seen in him as an infant continued, and other alarming conditions and behaviors began to emerge, all signs of *autism*.

Autism is a highly complex, neurodevelopmental disorder considered incurable by Western medicine. It is characterized by impairments in social interaction, communication, and behavior. Jacob had identified issues in each of those three areas, as well as sensory processing, metabolic, and gastrointestinal issues. In order to convey Jacob's healing from such a debilitating disability, I need to briefly relate his issues first.

Jacob was both sensory *avoidant* and sensory *seeking*. Although he sought out oral stimulation using objects and his own fingers, he was repulsed by many food textures. And although certain sounds caused him to clap his hands over his ears and collapse on the floor, he would turn up the volume on the television to an ear-splitting level. He also recoiled from the tactile feel of certain clothing, yet handled toys and furniture so roughly that he broke them. Jacob also reacted with violent tantrums to the slightest change in his routine. Transitions from awake to sleep, or from one activity to another, would also cause a "meltdown"— screaming that could last for hours.

Jacob's ability to communicate was severely impacted by three different diagnosed conditions seen in children with autism, specifically echolalia, apraxia of speech, and auditory processing disorder. He was unable to create novel speech other than the use of single words for family members or to indicate his desire for a specific food or toy. The rest of his speech consisted of parroting back whatever we said to him and phrases he heard on television or his movies—which he would repeat out of context throughout the day. Jacob also had difficulty with motor planning, the carrying out of purposeful movements necessary for speech. He was unable to process or appropriately respond to even the simplest of yes or no questions, and didn't seem to understand much of what was said to him.

Jacob had other conditions to be dealt with, metabolic difficulties and "leaky gut syndrome," an abnormal permeability of the intestinal wall that allows toxins and waste matter to leak into the circulatory system. This gastrointestinal disturbance is another of many conditions associated with vaccinations and autism.

To play, Jacob preferred to lie on his side with his head resting on the floor, due to muscle weakness. He would fixate on the wheels of his toy cars, a classic sign of autism. I read his thoughts and moods by observing his body language and using my mother's intuition... but that wouldn't help him connect with the outside world.

Once he became mobile, all the doors in our home had to be latched above his reach in order to keep Jacob safe, as he compulsively searched for a way to get out. Because of this wandering behavior, and his violent reactions that resulted from his difficulty processing sensory information, I was unable to take him anywhere outside the home. Store environments overwhelmed him and people would glare at me during his public outbursts. I became housebound.

My recurrent dreams during this time were of being under house arrest—a mirror of the reality of my life. As the body is considered a "house" for the spirit, the house in the dream was a metaphor for my body. The dreams were providing clues as to the state of my energy systems, which were being impacted by the daily trauma of Jacob's issues, effectively closing and locking the "doors" and "windows" of my "house." And I was unable to get any help to heal these developing energetic disruptions, because I couldn't find anyone willing to watch my high-need toddler in order to get to appointments.

Diagnosis?

At this point in a typical autism story, parents usually relate the time their child was diagnosed. Despite the severity of Jacob's disabilities, that day never came. The first time I heard the word autism in connection with Jacob was several years later, during a meeting with his special education teacher. While the school system professionals were deeply concerned about Jacob's communication difficulties and developmental delays, his rigidness, limited social skills, and muscle weakness—his pediatricians were not. The teacher urged us to pursue a definitive diagnosis.

The physicians who examined Jacob did not acknowledge his developmental delays, even when he consistently failed the office developmental questionnaire at each well check-up. No referrals were made and we were advised to "stop looking for problems" with our son and were sent on our way. Only years later would a pediatrician admit that Jacob's early difficulties were consistent with autism. But by the time we received that acknowledgment, it was too late for critical early intervention had we not already proceeded on our own to seek additional support and services.

In Western medicine, a diagnosis is very important. A diagnostic label is required in order to determine which drugs to use, and for insurance coverage. However, one does not need a Western medical diagnosis to receive services in natural healing systems. In fact, a diagnosis can be rather meaningless, as illness and disease states have the same origin—disturbed energy flow.

Jacob did not need a diagnosis of autism to receive physical, occupational, or speech therapy for his developmental delays, which he received for years. While these therapies were vital to his continued development, correcting the blockages in his energy systems for complete healing would require going outside of Western medicine, which didn't require a diagnosis either. We also didn't need a diagnosis to see a nutritionist who made a gluten-free, casein-free diet recommendation and suggested nutritional supplements to compensate for the poor absorption and digestion of nutrients from leaky-gut syndrome. While the supplements and diet recommendations were vital, ultimately he would heal the need for them.

I now see the benefit of our pediatricians' non-acknowledgment of Jacob's difficulties. If they had, he would have received a label considered incurable. Rather than being unduly influenced by a rather hopeless diagnosis, their lack of support just made it clear that Jacob's path to healing was not through Western medicine.

I have since learned that our experiences were not unusual. Even when a diagnosis of autism is made, most pediatricians and pediatric neurologists do not recommend anything other than behavioral therapy, such as Applied Behavior Analysis, or ABA therapy. Although many parents have found ABA therapy helpful for their children, it does not address the energy disruptions at the root cause of autism.

In addition to behavioral therapy, treatment can also be found through a DAN (Defeat Autism Now) physician. The DAN protocol consists of individualized diet and supplement recommendations, various methods of heavy metal chelation, and treatment for overgrowth of bacteria, yeast, and parasites. Although there are some risks associated with chelation treatment, the DAN protocol can achieve dramatic results.

I had been practicing as an energy healing practitioner years before I had Jacob, but his arrival in my life opened the door to a whole new level of understanding of healing. With no diagnosis, there was no referral for behavioral therapy or the DAN protocol. Instead, I turned my attention to finding help that would address the root of Jacob's issues, the disturbances in his energy systems. And in that search, I was referred to a healing practitioner who worked with quantum formulas, a type of vibrational medicine.

Through quantum formulas, Jacob's remarkable and complete recovery would be facilitated by achieving the same healing goals of heavy metal removal and correction of overgrowth of pathogens as the DAN protocol, and much more—all with no side effects and no risks. And even if we had been offered behavioral therapy, it became unnecessary because Jacob's behavioral issues resolved from the core with quantum formulas, although we did need to teach him appropriate behavior that did not come naturally to him.

Through my experiences with vibrational medicine, the preparation for my work in the world would deepen through an experiential education in more laws of healing.

Vibrational Medicine

Vibrational medicine is a therapeutic approach to health issues based on the premise that the essence of life is energy. Vibrational medicine includes "remedies" in such forms as flower essences, homeopathy, and quantum formulas.

Flower Essences

The original and most well-known of the flower essences were developed by Dr. Edward Bach, a London physician frustrated with conventional medicine. In 1930 he closed his lucrative medical practice and set off to find a new system of healing involving plants.

Dr. Bach discovered that the intake of high vibrational substances, such as plants and flowers, can raise low vibrational frequencies and positively impact health. Following this initial discovery, he determined how to transfer the vibrations of plants into water. By infusing spring water with wildflowers, either by "sun-steeping" or boiling, he created Bach Flower Remedies. Millions have benefited from these remedies over the last 75 years. Although their use has not yet become mainstream in the U.S. as they are in Europe, Bach Flower Remedies can be found in many American stores. References to flower essences have also made their way into popular television shows. In recent years more organizations have created flower essences, including the Perelandra Center for Nature Research in Jeffersonton, Virginia, and Green Hope Farm in Meriden, New Hampshire.

Homeopathy

Homeopathy is a healing system discovered by German physician Dr. Samuel Hahnemann in the early 1800s when he became disillusioned with "heroic" medicine, which was the practice at the time. Homeopathy is based on the law of similars, or "like is cured by like." In other words, if your illness symptoms are similar to the symptoms of mercury poisoning, then you would take the homeopathic remedy mercury.

Homeopathic remedies are prepared by diluting a substance at a ratio of 1:99 while striking the solution against an elastic body in a procedure known as "succussion." Paradoxically, the more times a remedy is diluted by this ratio, the more potent the healing action. At high dilutions, none of the original substance remains in the solution. Rather, only the frequency of the substance remains.

This is a peculiar concept for Western medicine, how a vial of water that appears to contain "nothing" can heal. In homeopathic philosophy, substances do not create healing. Rather, the *frequency* of substances *activates* healing. The high dilution of toxic medicinal substances in homeopathy creates effective agents of healing, safe and free of side effects.

In classical homeopathy, an individual's constitutional type is identified through a series of questions that determine patterns of physical, mental, emotional, behavioral, and illness response characteristics. Two individuals experiencing the same infectious illness could take different homeopathic remedies based on their constitutional type. Their constitutional remedy would stimulate their own individual, inner healing force.

Considered mainstream medical care in Europe, the use of homeopathy is gradually spreading in the United States, though nowhere near the extent of use seen prior to the publication of the Flexner Report in 1910.

Quantum Formulas

There are many different types of vibrational remedies used for healing, some formulated by organizations and some by individuals. The specific type used to facilitate Jacob's recovery was called "quantum formulas," made by the Healers Who Share organization in Denver, Colorado. In chapter 2 we learned that vibrational medicine works through destructive interference, the process of disintegrating vibrational frequencies that occurs when an out-of-sync wave cancels the wave of a pathogen, cancerous cell, or toxin. Similar to flower essences and homeopathy, quantum formulas come in the form of a vial of water containing a frequency.

No expensive lab testing is required for quantum formulas. To determine which vibrational remedy would cancel the frequencies of your particular issues, all that is needed is a cotton ball that has been swabbed inside your mouth to obtain saliva for energy analysis. You may recall the U.S. Army experiment from chapter 8, in which DNA separated from its donor source responded as if still one with the donor, regardless of the distance of that separation. Your saliva contains your DNA, which contains your energetic frequencies, as would any cell of your body, and can be sent any distance for energy analysis.

In chapter 9, we learned how telling a "lie" dramatically disrupts energy flow. For a healing practitioner having high coherence with the universal energy field, posing a series of yes or no questions, or true or false statements in the presence of donor DNA will separate "truth" from "lie" through a brief disruption in energy that the healing practitioner can detect in their own body as muscle weakness. For example, in the presence of a cotton ball with saliva DNA, a healing practitioner might begin with a statement such as, "The client's symptoms are related to a pathogen." If this is a "lie," the practitioner will detect a disruption of energy as muscle weakness. If this statement is true, there will be no energetic disruption, and further questions can be posed to determine if the pathogen is fungal, viral, bacterial, yeast, or parasitic in nature. Depending on the answers received, the next round of questions would pinpoint the specific pathogens involved, and which remedy would address the condition. We will discuss the use of muscle testing for energy analysis in more detail in chapter 14.

In Western medicine, testing for pathogens involves detecting their actual presence in bodily tissues and fluids. After such determination, a biochemical drug is used to eradicate the pathogen presence. However, the use of biochemical drugs does not address the underlying energetic condition that caused the pathogen to proliferate, nor can biochemical drugs address any of the associated physical, emotional, mental, or spiritual effects of the energetic condition. In fact, biochemical drugs can actually disturb body biochemistry and destroy beneficial pathogens.

Along with quantum formulas that targeted subclinical fungal, viral, bacterial, yeast, and parasitic infections, Jacob also took quantum formulas to address the many conditions associated with autism. He received quantum remedies formulated to cancel the vibrational frequency of mercury, a highly toxic heavy metal used as a preservative in many vaccinations and one of the suspected culprits in many cases of autism. Jacob also received formulas targeted to dismantle the frequencies underlying his severe difficulties with auditory processing, motor planning, hyperactivity, sensory integration disorder, leaky gut syndrome, and metabolic disorder.

After beginning quantum formulas, Jacob's impatience, irritability, frustration, rigidity and hyperactivity began to melt away. His issues with processing sensory information gradually resolved, and his ability to communicate and interact socially steadily improved. His tantrums decreased in number and severity until they stopped altogether. By age six, his remaining issues measured below the diagnostic standard on the autism scale administered by a school psychologist. However, there was still a developmental gap in all measured areas between him and his peers.

Six months later, that gap vanished almost overnight.

At six-and-a-half-years old, the muscle weakness that had made it difficult for Jacob to grasp a pencil or hold his head up while playing on the floor disappeared, as well as his need for supportive ankle braces. Although he was expected to require occupational and physical therapy for the foreseeable future, his startled therapists discharged him when all his recently set, long-term goals were met. His private speech therapist followed suit shortly thereafter, puzzled by Jacob's sudden developmental leap in language processing and communication skills. What had happened?

Jacob had experienced a *quantum leap* in healing. When a single possibility *actualizes*, which in Jacob's case was the possibility of collapsing the developmental gap, the waves of all other possibilities abruptly disintegrate. In that moment, all other possibilities cease to exist. In physics, this sudden leap from one state to another without any discernible process in between is referred to as a "quantum jump." A quantum jump is by its nature unpredictable and *unexpected*.

Healing Continues

My story about Jacob brings us to another principle of healing. Once established, the healing process will continue *unless further insult or obstruction takes place*.

At the time that it felt right to discontinue vibrational remedies for Jacob, he still had some subtle difficulties with conversational skills. Later that year, as I observed him in school during a party, there was noticeable improvement in his communication skills. Yet he had not received any healing therapies in six months. I wondered how he could still be healing without intervention.

As healing is a natural process, once it is established it will continue unless obstructed, as in the case of new trauma. Healing therapies work with the body's natural movement toward wholeness. Even when the therapy is discontinued, healing can continue if it was well-established.

Although I had released numerous blockages in my energy systems during the years of healing my infertility, that healing process became obstructed with the formation of new disturbances in my energy systems with Jacob's birth and his subsequent issues. His stay in the newborn intensive care unit had been traumatic for me, as were his severe difficulties with everyday life that overwhelmed our family during his early years. And Jacob's tremendous needs had made it difficult for me to attend to my own healing, or arrange child care assistance to obtain professional healing assistance for myself.

Worst of all was the lack of support from Jacob's pediatricians. I was on my own in navigating through both Western therapies and energy medicine therapies to find him help. But an accident I had when Jacob was fourteen months old would be the final blow to my already compromised energy systems, devastating my health.

While sewing and holding a straight pin between my lips, I inhaled sharply at the sight of Jacob's fingers dangerously close to the metal prongs of the sewing machine plug as he removed it from a wall outlet. With that intake of breath, the straight pin was pulled deep into my lung, necessitating major chest surgery to remove it.

Within months of this surgery, my health took a downward spiral. I relapsed into chronic fatigue syndrome and my blood sugar became so unstable I would feel faint every hour or two throughout the day. I also began gaining weight at an alarming rate. Under the grip of fatigue and all-day migraines, I passed the days on the couch while Jacob played nearby with his toys, in my house locked from the inside to keep him safe.

Just as healing has momentum, so can illness. Our energy systems become compromised from each traumatic encounter, until a critical point is reached where functioning is severely impacted.

If I had been able to receive healing therapies in a timely manner to correct the energy blockages and imbalances created by the surgery, the health crisis would likely have been averted. I once saw a craniosacral therapist, but was unable to continue. Given that Jacob screamed the entire time I was gone for that one appointment, the lady who cared for him in my absence refused to ever watch him again.

Regardless of the lack of child care, I had to find a way to recover. The healing practitioner who worked effectively with Jacob through the use of energy-based healing therapies and quantum formulas became the perfect solution. Once again, it seemed that Jacob was leading me by example. As I witnessed his recovery, I knew that energy healing and quantum formulas were the answer for me as well, and I could bring him along to my appointments.

Hering's Second Law of Cure

As I recovered, my healing proceeded according to the second rule of Hering's Law of Cure, which states that healing progresses in the reverse order from which it began. The very first symptom of illness in my life began when I was a teenager—chronic sinus infections. As I healed with vibrational remedies, over several months I re-experienced in reverse order every stage of illness throughout my life, ending with a final sinus infection. However, each re-occurrence was only a fraction of the time of the original illness.

That final infection was different than the sinus infections I had experienced for decades. Those left me feeling weak and depleted, requiring recovery time. In contrast, when this last infection resolved I felt energized and invigorated. Since then, I haven't had a single sinus infection in over ten years, which is amazing considering I had four to six infections every year for twenty-five years.

Today Jacob is a vibrant, engaging, well-spoken, and athletic young man who adapts to change easily. He assimilates auditory information competently and has no memory of being disabled. People who meet him now have no idea that he once had all the characteristics of autism. His presence serves as a daily reminder that miracles do happen. I continue to learn from him, and to this day, he continues to heal.

As recovery from autism is generally not considered within the realm of possibilities by many Western medical professionals, our pediatrician's only explanation for his recovery is that he must not have had autism in the first place, as if the disabling conditions identified by the many professionals who worked with Jacob never existed.

Since my experience with Jacob, I have come to recognize spiritual partnerships with all my children, my husband, and other people in my life. Every client who walks through my office door brings situations that teach me. The writing of this book has been accomplished through spiritual partnerships. Whenever I was missing an example for a concept, or needed a deeper understanding, it would appear in my life—whether through my personal relationships, clients in my practice, or even my dogs!

I now realize that we are *all* interacting on a spiritual level, as we are all connected to each other. This energetic dynamic is at work even when such connections create trauma. The pediatricians who did not support me were interacting on a spiritual level by mirroring back victim frequency, although I did not recognize it at the time.

So we see that trauma creates an *opportunity*. When we heal from a traumatic event, that healing can become *globalized,* unwinding the negative belief patterns that create layers of energy blockages. This is the experience of *transformation.* My infertility trauma became the opportunity to heal childhood wounds, unraveling the negative belief patterns formed early in life and releasing layers of energy system blockages back to their source. Moreover, the trauma related to Jacob's early childhood became the opportunity to heal more layers of those old wounds.

Hering's Third Law of Cure

There is one more of Hering's principles to examine: the third law, which states that healing progresses from the upper part of the body to the lower part. Energy blocks often release according to Hering's first or third law of cure, either from the inside of the body to the outside, or from the upper part of the body to the lower part. Thousands of times in my own healing and that of my clients, I have witnessed Hering's third law of cure at work in directing the release of energy blockages, which move down the body and out the feet unless there is a second block lower in the body that interrupts the flow of the release.

Audrey had suffered two miscarriages, the first one an

unplanned pregnancy two months after she got married and the second a year later. She had been recently plagued with depression, lower back pain, "nervous" stomach, and difficulty taking in a deep breath. As Audrey described the mixed feelings she had when she discovered she was pregnant so soon after her wedding, her energy rhythms changed and became disharmonious. At the same time that I perceived this change in her vibration, Audrey reported an increase in the anxious sensation in her abdomen.

I encouraged Audrey to breathe into the anxious sensation as she expressed regret over her ambivalence with her first pregnancy—a regret deepened with the loss of that pregnancy, and also the next. As she described her guilt, Audrey burst into tears. With her tears, she felt the release of the anxious sensation in her stomach as it moved down her body and out her feet.

As Audrey experienced the release of the energy blockage, my hand was resting on her abdomen and I felt a sensation of sudden movement at the same time. With that movement of energy, Audrey spontaneously took in a deep breath and then relaxed, saying, "I had no idea that I still had such guilt and sadness over something that happened over a year ago."

The movement of an energy release can also follow Hering's first law of cure, from the inside to the outside of the body, or along an acupuncture meridian.

If tendonitis of the elbow becomes tendonitis of the wrist and then the hand, one might think the condition is only getting worse. However, this progression of symptoms further away from the core of the body is an encouraging sign of healing. Such a progression can occur if the inflammation is managed through natural means such as ice, heat, manipulation, and an anti-inflammatory diet of raw vegetables and fruit.

In cases of suppression, we see "violations" of Hering's laws of cure with a progression of symptoms that are opposite of the expected course of healing. Tess had chronic inflammatory pain in her knee. She explained that she had "healed" inflammation in her Achilles tendon in the past with over-the-counter anti-inflammatory medication and injections of cortisone from her physician. But now she had inflammation in her knee that was even worse than the Achilles tendon inflammation had been. Her physician recommended higher doses of anti-inflammatory medication, but Tess sought a more natural approach.

Although Tess's Achilles tendon pain had previously subsided, it hadn't actually healed. The suppressed inflammation had simply moved from lower in the body to higher, a violation of Hering's third law of cure.

Even though I had worked with clients like Tess—and was well aware of the consequences of using anti-inflammatory medication to treat inflammation—when experiencing inflammation of my own knee, I could not resist the temptation to use medication to speed up the resolution. Within a few days the knee inflammation did indeed resolve, but a week later, my hip on the same side became inflamed and swollen, impinging upon lower back nerves and causing severe pain. One might think these were two separate issues, but in fact the inflammation of the knee did not heal. It had only been driven further toward the core of my body.

I hope these stories will inspire you to follow your own path to healing, in whatever form it may take. As we have seen, a healing story can encompass any life experience or modality, including both Western medicine and energy medicine. In the next chapter, we will examine additional principles as signs to follow on the journey of healing.

Even though I may react to or be triggered by others, I recognize these occurrences as a mirror of my own energetic frequencies and I send love and acceptance to where I am wounded.

Even though I may have been traumatized by others, I recognize the role they have played in my healing, and I love and accept myself. I trust in the divine wisdom evident in the laws that govern that healing, and allow my process to unfold naturally.

~ 13 ~

HEALING SIGNS

*"Endings and beginnings, with emptiness and germination
in between. That basic shape is so essential to growth that
we must learn to recognize it in our lives."*

— WILLIAM BRIDGES

IMAGINE YOU HAVE followed the steps of healing—become more aware and self-compassionate, built trust with yourself, and have been able to let go.

Now...what should you expect? How do you know you are healing? If you've never been there, how do you recognize it?

Here are some of the changes my clients have reported:

- Vibrations, particularly in the hands and feet
- Increased awareness of environment, body, or emotions
- Body feels different
- Respond to situations differently
- Acting differently in dream life
- Emotional ups and downs are more shallow
- Less occupied with the past or the future

- More in the moment
- Changes in relationships and relating to others
- Improved health
- Improved mental clarity and focus
- Increased energy
- Changes in beliefs
- Changes in lifestyle
- New understanding of old situations
- Sense of well-being
- Increased confidence
- Reduced stress and increased relaxation
- Cessation of addictive patterns
- Experiences of synchronicity
- Seeing colors around people or animals

Sometimes the people in our lives will recognize the changes in us more quickly than we do. Here are some of the comments my clients have reported from others:

- "There's something different about you."
- "You are just glowing. What's going on?"
- "You look like a weight has been lifted off your shoulders."
- "You seem so relaxed."
- "I've never seen you like this before."

Let's take a more detailed look at a few of these changes.

Increased Awareness

As I became engaged in my healing process, I had a number of experiences that indicated I was healing. The first was increased awareness of my body.

One particular day I was startled to find that the simple, everyday act of taking a shower was entirely different. I was suddenly aware of the wonderful sensation of warm water flowing over my skin, as if I was experiencing it for the first time. The smell of the shampoo filled my senses as I took in a full, deep breath and massaged it into my scalp. How could I have never noticed how good it felt just to take a shower and wash my hair? It was an act of daily living I had robotically performed thousands of times, a simple daily pleasure suddenly available by being fully present in the moment.

I also noticed moments when everything in my environment seemed brighter and clearer. Colors appeared sharper. It was as if I had been wearing sunglasses and had just taken them off.

In addition to becoming more aware, my body just felt "different." One aspect of my energy system dysfunction had been the absence of energy flow through my legs. As that energy flow resumed, the sensation felt odd. Initially, my legs felt literally as big as an elephant's. But it wasn't long before the sensation of energy flow through my legs felt normal, and I no longer perceived my leg size as being usually large.

During this time of increased awareness, the nurses on the unit where I worked began behaving differently toward me. As I arrived for work, my colleagues would exclaim, "You're here!" or "It's you!"

"Um, yeah, I'm here....it's me. But what's with the celebrity treatment?" I asked.

"You're like a breath of fresh air. It's as if the whole room lights up when you're here!"

The first time I ever used Emotional Freedom Technique (EFT), a self-help method of energy medicine that involves tapping on acupoints, I worked through some issues of poor body image due to my excess weight. Using a protocol I found on the

Internet, I tapped while reading statements about loving my body and appreciating its function. After I finished my tapping session, I went to a birthday party where there was a large spread of food. Normally, I would have become more focused on the food than the people, resulting in mentally obsessing about the food and overeating.

However, on this day, just after acutapping, strangely I was not drawn to the food at all. When offered cake, I easily declined. But the most unusual aspect of the day was the comments from others. Three different people exclaimed how good I looked and wanted to know what was different about me—A new haircut? New clothes? A weight loss?

What change in me had both my work colleagues and the guests at the party noticed? When energy blockages release and the flow of energy is restored, the result is a noticeable increase in vibrational frequency that we perceive as radiance and attractiveness.

Changes in Relationships

As she healed, Rita noticed that she no longer became reactive to certain situations. In the past, if her husband told her she was being stubborn, or her sister told her she was being selfish, she would become defensive. Now in the process of healing, Rita feels no angst in response to these statements from her loved ones. As she has brought these aspects of herself out of the shadow and into acceptance, the comments of others are no longer perceived as criticisms. This is the experience of being centered and anchored in your authentic core self.

Imagine two upright bowling pins, one resting on the floor unanchored, and the other anchored to the floor and the ceiling by a vertical cord through a drilled center. If you roll a bowling ball at the unanchored pin, it will be easily knocked over. If you roll a bowling ball at the anchored pin, it will remain grounded through its core connections. In this analogy, the floor represents the Earth and the ceiling the universal energy field. The unanchored pin represents an individual oriented to ego, and the bowling ball those situations, criticisms, and hurts that usually knock us over. When you are connected to the universal energy field and grounded in the truth of who you are, the "bowling balls of life" will no longer knock you over because you know to your core that you are a worthy and loveable person regardless. When you are centered in your core, you are able to recognize your value as the *truth,* and any devaluing situations, thoughts, or words as *false.*

Tess's healing process had included healing her inner critical "judge." As she developed self-compassion and her relationship with herself changed, Tess began feeling less critical of her adult children. As her self-judging frequencies shifted to self-acceptance, her adult children were suddenly attracted back into her life, after months of absence.

Not all reactions from others to the shifts produced by healing are complimentary and supportive. The movement of energy can create both positive and negative changes in relationships. Here are some examples of comments clients have reported hearing from others.

- "What's wrong with you?"
- "I can't figure you out."
- "You aren't fun anymore."

When one person in a relationship changes, the other is automatically affected. Depending on the situation, that effect may or may not be considered desirable. With a shift in energetic frequency, some relationships will flourish and some will flounder. Others will go through a period of growing pains as adjustments are made.

Throughout Vanessa's marriage, her need to be a victim was fulfilled by her husband's need to rescue her. When she began healing the victim, he felt lost.

"He says he just wants us to go back to the way we were," Vanessa lamented. "But I can't ever go back. I'm not that young, troubled girl he married. This is the real me now."

In social situations, people who you thought were "fun" may now seem dysfunctional. Or people may think *you* are no longer fun because you aren't validating the stories they have made up about themselves, or are no longer participating in formerly shared activities such as drinking alcohol or judging others through gossip. It may become difficult to be around people who are inauthentic, because when you become authentic, you vibrate to a different frequency. These people may now seem "fake" or superficial. But even so, if they do leave your life, you may feel very alone and afraid that you will not meet someone new who is more "in sync" with you.

It was at this stage of healing that Vanessa made blanket statements about others, saying "everyone" was superficial and that she didn't fit in with "anyone." This was likely true, as everyone in her current life resonated with her previous state of energy system blockages. As she healed the disturbances in her energy systems, Vanessa no longer had coherence with her friends. The people in our lives are a reflection of the predominant state of our energy.

On an energetic level, these changes in relationships may have you feeling like you no longer speak the same "language." Or you may have a "falling out" with someone close to you, meaning you are no longer "in sync" with that person. With that loss of synchronicity, you may no longer share the same viewpoints, or worse yet, you may actually feel drained from contact with them.

Although sometimes relationships do end in the process of healing, this should not be taken lightly, as social support is vital to health. In the next chapter we will discuss the energetic nature of relationships in greater detail, along with guidelines for navigating the difficulties and opportunities that relationships can present for healing.

Synchronicity

When resistance is removed and blockages are released, energy flow is restored and synchronicities can begin to happen, sometimes immediately. At the end of an appointment, it is my custom to offer clients the opportunity to randomly select and read a card from a deck, such as Louise Hay's *Wisdom Cards*. These cards serve as a divination tool, similar to a pendulum or dousing rod. Often the card a client pulls is a precise match for the intuitive messages that came through during that day's session to help with the client's particular issues. In this way, the cards deepen the healing. However, these occurrences can lead some clients to believe I am a magician! While they may seem like magic, synchronicities are quantum physics at work.

Clients report other synchronicities, such as seeing a license plate or a particular road sign on the drive home that contains words, phrases, or numbers that seem too much of a coincidence, or they will make sudden connections through chance encounters or unexpected phone calls. Jim had not had any contact from his mother or his mother's extended family for decades. He felt alone and abandoned, but believed that reconnecting with his lost family was impossible. After one of our sessions, Jim received an email from a member of his mother's family who had tracked him down. They subsequently had a joyful reunion.

As the healing process progresses, these moments of synchronicity can increase in frequency, becoming daily occurrences. These synchronicities happen when we become aligned with our spiritual connection to the universal energy field, experiences that many attribute to angels and the presence of God.

Am I Healing...OR NOT?

Perhaps you aren't experiencing these changes or synchronicities, or only experienced them temporarily and now feel stuck. Or you might think your issues are actually worse. What might be happening? These situations could be caused by one of two scenarios—your healing process has stalled, or you are having difficulty recognizing the process of healing, because progress may not seem like progress.

If no changes have taken place or you feel stuck, it may come as no surprise that the factors that cause blockages in our energy systems are the same factors that can block the healing process: *beliefs, resistance,* and *suppression.*

Here are some of the beliefs that prevent people from getting better:

- "If I get better, something will be expected of me."
- "If I get better, I'm just setting myself up for failure when I get sick again."
- "As long as I'm sick, I can stay in the same place, which feels safe."
- "If I get better, people won't take care of me anymore."
- "If I change, people will reject and abandon me."

You may notice that each of those beliefs is based on fears, and not surprisingly, those fears are usually formed from traumatic experiences such as attachment trauma and misuse of power. Childhood trauma can result in the belief that love and acceptance have to be earned through performance.

Nora's issues began after her brother's death and progressively got worse. She was unhappy, depressed, and suffered from a pervasive sense of inertia as her energy was caught up in her compulsions. During a healing therapy session, Nora suddenly realized that, deep down, she didn't want to get better because if she did it would be a "dishonor" to her brother. Since her brother didn't get to live, she felt she wasn't entitled to be happy and healthy. This realization came as quite a shock to her.

Rita had a more unusual belief that blocked her healing, stemming from traumatic encounters with the Western medical community. She felt she wasn't being heard or taken seriously by the physicians she consulted. Rita admitted that when it came to allopathic professionals, her inner dialogue went something like this: "I'll show you! I won't respond to your treatment. In fact, I'll get even worse, and then maybe you'll take me seriously and really hear me!" Although this may sound irrational, any response to trauma is *valid*. Once we become aware of the beliefs that are blocking our healing, we can feel compassion for the wounded places within, from which this belief was formed—and choose acceptance. For Rita, healing this block was about fulfilling her unmet need to be heard. By seriously considering her seemingly irrational response and allowing herself to fully express her hurt and frustration, the block was released and her healing process resumed.

Sometimes people don't heal because they are attached to a

specific outcome, or to achieving that outcome in a specific way. Or they think they've let go, but really haven't. Others don't heal because they are not allowing the expression of their emotions or are using other suppressive means to manage their illness.

Attachment to outcome creates resistance to other possibilities and is a form of control. You may recall that my attachment to the manner in which my infertility was to resolve had stalled my healing process and blocked resolution. Learning this principle of healing through the infertility experience proved valuable when faced with Jacob's issues. After compassionately allowing myself to fully express how overwhelmed I was, I meditated on the feeling of already having the help for Jacob that I desperately needed, while letting go of what form that help would take, as well as when it would arrive.

As an aid in healing, I used the ancient Chinese study of the movement of energy in one's environment, known as *Feng Shui*. From quantum physics we know that everything is energy, including our environment. Our homes can be just as much a mirror of our inner energy as the people in our lives. Areas of our home that are cluttered or in a state of disrepair can be a reflection of discord in areas of our lives. As such, rearranging our home environment can create changes in our health, happiness, and relationships.

When I considered the nine areas of the bagua, the Feng Shui energy map of any given space, in terms of Jacob's needs, I knew I should focus on the "helpful friends" area. After de-cluttering this area, I considered what might represent the help I desired. What came to mind was an image of Mary Poppins, a character in a Walt Disney film of the same name, who magically arrived in a household in need of care for the children. I placed an old movie poster that featured an image of Mary Poppins in the helpful friends area of our bedroom with the intention and expectation of help for Jacob, as if it had already arrived.

It wasn't long before Jacob qualified for special education preschool in our county. As I had envisioned, he was getting the help he needed, and with that I regained balance in my life. Mary Poppins had indeed arrived!

Fear of Power

Ultimately a block in the healing process can be caused by an unconscious fear of our own *power*. Most of the traumas discussed in this book resulted from a misuse of power. If you have been the victim of misuse of power in childhood, relationships, jobs, organizations, religions, or medical systems that involve the use of force, especially in cases of physical, emotional, mental, spiritual, and sexual abuse, you may fear having power yourself. And in order to prevent ourselves from becoming powerful, we can unconsciously block our healing by using force against ourselves in the form of self-rejecting thoughts and actions, such as suppressing our emotions and dismissing our intuition. These negative thoughts and actions effectively disengage us from our own power and the responsibilities that come with it.

In *Power Vs Force: The Hidden Determinants of Human Behavior,* David Hawkins, M.D., Ph.D. has developed a scale of human consciousness that sheds light on the true meaning of power. As I have touched on in earlier chapters, the consciousness states of shame, guilt, apathy, grief, fear, desire, anger, and pride are all associated with low vibrational frequencies, an absence of spirituality, weakness, and the use of *force*. It is when this force is used against us that trauma is created, resulting in mistrust and misuse of power. But it is important to note that what we fear is actually the use of force associated with *powerless* states, not power.

True, authentic power is an expression of the high vibrational consciousness states of courage, neutrality, willingness, acceptance, unconditional love, peace, and grace. It is in these states that spirituality enters the picture. Authentic power is never forceful. Rather, it is a high- frequency state associated with physical, emotional, mental, and spiritual strength that comes through us, not from us, when our consciousness and vibrational level rise through alignment with our core, authentic selves. To enter this realm of authentic power, all we need is courage to begin to rise above shame, guilt, apathy, grief, fear, desire, anger, and pride.

For many of my clients, especially women, this erroneous belief that power is synonymous with the use of force can create a situation where they unconsciously choose disease and illness over personal power. Individuals who have been traumatized by the use of force through sexual abuse, religious doctrine, aggressive medical treatment, or any situation marked by manipulation, control, coercion, narcissism, judgment, arrogance, or rejection— are *loath* to claim their own power out of fear that they will also use force like the individuals and institutions that have traumatized them. Instead they use force against themselves.

I want to note here that sometimes forceful action is necessary in acute, life-threatening situations, such as resetting a compound fracture or pulling a child back from running into traffic. But the route to authentic healing is always unconditional acceptance through patience and gentleness. For example, when I encounter a stuck cranial bone during a healing session that is causing the client a headache and diminished function, any use of force will engage the body's natural reaction to protect itself through resistance, and will fail to effect change. It is through letting go of how, when, and even *if* the bone will move, and by holding it in unconditional patience and gentleness—trusting in the divine wisdom present in the energy systems of the individual and their natural ability to heal—that the cranial bone can regain its mobility. Paradoxically, having no attachment to how long healing will take and accepting its natural timetable can actually speed up the process.

As with the healing of a cranial bone, so it is with life. No matter what your physical, emotional, mental, or spiritual issues are, the use of force against yourself, or the use of forceful systems to create change, will ultimately fail.

For those who have blocked their healing due to a fear of misuse of power, it is important to note that the misuse of power includes *not* using your power. When we block our healing process by disengaging from our power through staying caught up in whatever life circumstance is creating the block in our energy, we are aligned with our ego-selves and are in victim consciousness. In this situation we have taken ourselves out of the flow of the universe. We have removed ourselves from love. We have disengaged from our life purpose. We have shirked our responsibilities. And we have kept our gifts from others. As discussed throughout this book, the "treatment" for this affliction is *love*—unconditional love and acceptance of every part of us, including the fearful parts, and the parts that want to disengage.

Active Participation Required

Sometimes our healing process becomes blocked through resistance because we are not ready for the inner work, upheaval, and commitment required for healing. It may be easier to stay where you are—and that's a valid desire. Depending on the extent of your issues, the state of your energy systems, and the level of your resistance, the initial stage of the ongoing process of healing can be long and difficult.

I have had a number of clients come for one session with the assumption that seeing a healing therapist would be as passive as getting a massage. Once they realized that the process required their active participation, they didn't come back. A healing therapist is your personal consultant, but you are in charge and responsible for your own health. Some of these clients who were not ready at first came back years later, when their energy disturbances had progressed to a crisis situation.

In the film *The Matrix,* the character Cypher preferred to be inserted back into the matrix, even though he knew it was an illusion, because real life was too difficult. When contemplating his old life, which he knew was only an illusion, Cypher said, "Ignorance is bliss."

As we go through the mourning process of our old life, there may be times when we feel like Cypher, that we would prefer the illusion of the false self to the real world revealed once we become centered in who we are. In taking the red pill offered by Morpheus, Cypher woke up to reality, but he was not fully informed of what it would be like to become aware that his life as he knew it was only an illusion. Later in the film, Cypher speaks to the unconscious Morpheus, "If you had told us the truth, we would've told you to shove that red pill right up your ass."

The closer we get to the moment of release and surrender, the stronger the impulse to stop the process. This parallels the labor and birth process when some women voice *I can't do this*, just as the baby is about to be born. This parallel exists because healing *is* a birth process. But healing always happens in the right time. If we chose to halt our healing process, there will always be other opportunities.

Some people do choose to disengage from their healing process and go back to emotionally numbing practices, such as prescription medication, substance abuse, or consumption of sugar and processed foods. But usually these expressions of resistance and regret are passing thoughts that are a part of the grieving process. Allowing these thoughts and feelings to fully express without judgment opens the door for embracing your new life at higher frequencies.

Recognizing Healing

If your issues are progressing according to one or all of Hering's Laws of Cure, and you are experiencing some of the changes listed at the beginning of this chapter, you can be confident that healing is occurring. However, it is not always that easy to recognize.

Feeling whole can be a foreign concept when being unbalanced has become one's natural state. Sometimes we are living in a state of energy systems are so *off*-balance we have no idea what it feels like to *be* balanced.

After weeks, months, years, or perhaps decades of being addicted to the adrenalin rush of stress and anxiety, one might expect a similarly hyped-up, super-charged experience of healing. But the feeling of deep peace and well-being that comes with healing is not necessarily fireworks. This may come as quite a surprise for some, and even be perceived as boring. If you are in this stage, you may wonder—*this is it?*

It can take time to recognize the difference between an

adrenalin-fueled high and true joy. And until we recognize that difference, we may unconsciously fill our lives with more stress to restore the adrenal rush that feels missing. But after an adjustment period, that adrenaline rush can feel unnatural and toxic in comparison to the natural sense of bliss that the process of healing restores. Similarly, after we adjust to eating healthy foods, junk food and refined sugar can taste toxic and artificial as we recover our natural palate for whole and raw foods.

The "Apex" Problem

Sometimes when an issue is resolved through healing, the client doesn't notice its absence unless I bring it to their attention. We are much more likely to be aware of physical or emotional pain when it is present than when it is not. When I do bring it to the attention of my clients, they may pass off the change as "coincidence" and not attribute it to energy healing therapies.

This phenomenon of not crediting treatment with resolution is referred to as the "Apex Problem" by Thought Field Therapy founder Dr. Roger Callahan. This is a term he borrowed from British journalist Arthur Koestler and alludes to the mind not operating at its peak, or "apex." It is for this reason that I keep detailed notes of my sessions, including the client's numerical rating for their distress, using a scale of one to ten. This is to help determine the effectiveness of my work, and to assist clients in recognizing their healing.

Mandy was a young woman in the process of rebuilding her inner and outer life after a series of disappointing experiences that shook her sense of self to the core. A recent college graduate with student loan debt, she had taken any job she could get to pay her bills. But that job wasn't in alignment with her authentic self.

As we worked together, Mandy was having difficulty identifying healing.

"The last time you were here, you mentioned your stomach hurt every time you thought about quitting your job. How is that now?" I asked Mandy.

"I don't remember that," said Mandy, looking puzzled.

"According to my notes, you expressed significant ambivalence about this and rated your tension at an eight when we discussed it."

"I did?"

"Yes, we related it to the incident in your childhood when your family went bankrupt, and worked with that."

"That sounds familiar."

"Do you feel any tension right now while we are talking about this?"

"No. I feel fine. In fact, I did quit my job, even though I don't have a new one lined up yet."

"Wow, that's quite a change for you! Are you stressed about paying your bills? I know that's been a real issue for you in the past."

"No. That's what's so strange. I'm not stressed at all. I've been stretching more after my work-out routine, so maybe that's what's keeping me more relaxed."

"I'm sure the stretching is helpful, but I think there's more to it than that. Stretching in and of itself does not usually release an energy blockage. The fact that you got very tense at the moment you talked about quitting your job indicated there was a disturbance in your energy. And since you now indicate there is no tension related to this subject—that tells me that particular energy disturbance has been released."

"Perhaps," said Mandy.

This apex problem occurs when healing violates belief systems. Rather than changing a deeply held belief system, the mind searches for an explanation for the illogical. In the West, it is believed that physical, emotional, mental, and spiritual distress are relieved by allopathic, psychological, and religious systems of care through the use of biochemical drugs, talk therapy, or religious practices. While these treatments can certainly relieve symptoms, we generally do not accept that all our distressing issues on every level can be healed at the root cause with energy-based therapies. When faced with evidence that they do, the mind goes into denial.

While the apex problem can interfere with the recognition of healing, the nonlinear nature of healing itself can make it difficult to recognize as well. Because healing does not necessarily progress in a straight line, healing may not look like healing. We saw this phenomenon with Hering's Laws of Cures and other principles of healing discussed in previous chapters. Now we will examine several other nonlinear aspects of healing: the death, transition, and rebirth cycles, the spiral pattern, and the healing crisis.

When Progress Doesn't Look Like Progress

For decades, Vanessa unconsciously blocked herself from feeling the pain of her unhappy childhood. She likened herself to a robot, going through life performing tasks and staying very busy so she wouldn't have to feel her inner pain and could continue "holding it together." But once that façade began to crumble, she went through a stage where she no longer wanted to engage in any of her old activities. Eventually she stopped trying to hold it together and let go. This was followed by a time period lacking in motivation and with dreams that featured death themes.

Although Vanessa thought she had let go of everything, in fact she was still in resistance, resisting the loss of her old robotic way of life. It was difficult for her to believe that this could be progress. This is the stage before birthing a new life, the transition that occurs after the death of the old. This transition stage occurs when the old beliefs and ways of being are gone, but there is not yet anything new to replace it.

During this time one can feel confused, lost, and bewildered, as if the rug has been pulled out from under you—the dark night of the soul. The feelings of loss can come in waves, similar to the waves of contractions a woman in childbirth labor experiences—the work involved in the transition process. You may feel like you've just caught your breath and are starting to get a sense of stability when another wave hits. Trying to stay in the same place in the midst of change is like trying to be stationary on a boat in a storm. You may fear that you will drown. Or you may feel very empty inside because you have emptied out the old way of being. Resisting this stage can delay the beginning of the rebirth cycle.

It can be reassuring to know that when one cycle ends, another always begins. No storm lasts forever. The clouds will eventually clear and the sun will come out. The more we can let go of the old and trust that we will not drown in the waves of change, the sooner we will be out of the transition stage and into the time of rebirth.

Even when Vanessa was living with new beliefs and a new understanding of herself, she would still have occasional episodes of the old pain—anger, grief, and anxiety—which left her confused. Was she getting worse? Had her healing process stopped? Why was her emotional pain returning?

Vanessa was experiencing the *spiral* aspect of the healing

process. Healing follows a spiral pattern, circling and recycling as deeper and deeper layers of an issue are cleared and released. When this happens, it may feel like you are going backwards. You may wonder why an issue that you had thought was resolved is now "back." If you are re-experiencing an old issue, know that you are healing another *layer* or aspect of that issue. This is a sign that your healing is *deepening*, not stopping or going backwards.

As healing is the ongoing process of life, it is normal to experience many death, transition, and rebirth cycles during our lives, just as every year winter follows fall, and spring follows winter. We are continually being presented with opportunities to change, grow, and transform. When these opportunities are embraced rather than resisted, they provide fertile ground for growth. And as the process deepens, the duration of these cycles can accelerate, with resolution occurring as quickly as in a single day.

Healing Crisis

Rita called me early in her healing process, in a panic between sessions. She had come to me for anxiety, but now that anxiety was worse than ever.

"I seem to be having a relapse. I know the goal of healing therapies is to activate healing, but it doesn't seem to be working. How can I get the healing process started?" she asked.

I'm sure by now you know the answer for Rita as well as I do. Her healing process had indeed been activated. This re-experiencing of old symptoms that is seen in the patterns and laws that govern the healing process is referred to as a *healing crisis*.

A healing crisis is a natural occurrence in the course of healing. As energy systems open and clear, the toxic matter that accumulates as a result of energetic blockages, disruptions, and stagnation is released. The release of this toxic matter can cause symptoms on every level—physical, emotional, mental, and spiritual. One can experience flu-like symptoms, such as fever, fatigue, headache, joint aches, muscle pain, nausea, and diarrhea. The toxic negative beliefs and emotions that result from trauma can surface as they release, becoming more pronounced. In addition, repressed memories may be regained, spiritual beliefs may shift, and one's sense of identity may be shaken as the shadow story is shed.

This "house cleaning" that happens during a healing crisis generally only lasts a day or two, although it is sometimes longer. It is important to avoid suppressing symptoms and allow them to fully express while supporting the body through natural means.

In the next chapter we will examine the many ways one can activate and deepen the process of healing, and support ourselves through a healing crisis. I call these measures that are available to anyone at anytime *everyday energy medicine.*

Even though at times I feel I am getting worse or going backwards and lose faith in my healing process, I nurture myself with love and acceptance. I now recognize and embrace with gratitude the signs that I am healing.

Even though I may be afraid of abandonment and withdrawal of love and acceptance from others if I heal and change, I'm grounded in the knowledge that I am always completely loveable and cherished by the Divine, including my fears.

Even though I may be blocking my own healing through

my attachments, resistance, and fears, I am creating the trust within myself required to let go by loving and accepting myself unconditionally.

PART FOUR:

ENERGETIC SELF-CARE ESSENTIALS

HEALING PRACTICES THAT REALLY WORK

"The ultimate approach to healing will be to remove the abnormalities at the subtle-energy level which led to the manifestation of illness in the first place. This will be the greatest difference in approach between the traditional medicine of today and the spiritual/holistic medicine of the future."

—RICHARD GERBER, MD

~ 14 ~

THE HEALING WAY OF LIFE

Everyday Energy Medicine for
Your Body, Mind, and Spirit

"Live in rooms full of light
Avoid heavy food
Be moderate in the drinking of wine
Take massage, baths, exercise, and gymnastics
Fight insomnia with gentle rocking or the sound of running water
Change surroundings and take long journeys
Strictly avoid frightening ideas
Indulge in cheerful conversation and amusements
Listen to music."

—AULUS CORNELIUS CELSUS 25 B.C.E.—50 A.D.

AS A CHILD, the land where I lived was my playground. I road my bike on a dirt road, letting the leaves from the lower branches of the trees that lined the trail glide over my face. I swam in a pond under a 200-year-old oak tree, picked wild strawberries in a meadow, and gathered fresh vegetables from our garden. I climbed to the top of the hill, took in the view of the valley stretched out before me, and lay in the tall grass. In those moments, all seemed right with the world.

I eagerly anticipated the changes each season brought, and inwardly celebrated the ebb and flow of spring, summer, fall, and winter. The predictable rhythm of the seasons gave me a sense of stability, something I could count on when my home life felt so volatile. My attachment to the land gave me the comfort, security, and grounding that was missing in my life. Nature was salve to my troubled soul, providing sanctuary from my father's rage. To this day, I dream of my childhood nature playground, and go there in my mind when I need a moment of peace.

When my father's company transferred him to another region of the country, I was devastated. With the loss of my beloved nature sanctuary as a result of the move, I became deeply depressed. Separated from family, friends and acquaintances, I felt excruciatingly self-conscious amid strangers in my new high school. I began skipping meals and eating processed diet food in an effort to look more like the pictures in my teen magazines, and to gain acceptance with my new peers. When that failed to garner more friends, I retreated to my bedroom in our new home, where I spent so much of my remaining teen years.

Depriving myself of nature experiences, fresh air, and sunlight, I began to suffer from fatigue and chronic infections. So despite the traumas of my childhood, it wasn't until I stopped living in alignment with nature that my health began to suffer. And it wasn't until my early 30s that I became aware of the implications of this loss and took steps to correct the lack of nature in my life.

The self-care practices that I began to employ during that time of awakening signaled a return to nature. While sessions with a healing therapist and a psychotherapist were critical to my healing process, it was the natural self-care practices that I engaged in day-to-day that *integrated* that healing to my core.

In this final chapter, we will be examining these everyday ways that healing is available to all of us. As we explore these self-care practices that are elements of a healing way of life, we will be revisiting some of the characters in this book.

By self-care, I do not mean practices that conform to societal standards of beauty, such as the use of anti-wrinkle creams, unhealthy dieting practices, or cosmetic procedures. Rather, I am referring to self-care that is about loving and valuing your whole self—mind, body, and spirit. These self-help practices work with the energy systems of the body—increasing awareness, activating healing, promoting energetic vitality, and providing support through a healing crisis and the integration process. These natural measures are also helpful in preparing for, and recovering from, any necessary conventional medical treatment.

We have learned that the healing process begins with awareness and progresses through compassion, self-love, and self-acceptance. Love and acceptance of self *includes* nurturing ourselves through self-care measures that fulfill health needs, practices that I refer to as *everyday energy medicine.*

The Healing Power of Nature

The disconnection from nature that I experienced as a teenager has emerged as an alarming trend throughout the world in recent years—especially among the young—the result of decreasing access to shrinking natural spaces and shifts in public perception. Lives historically in harmony with nature have been replaced with a modern view of nature as dangerous and a force to be controlled and exploited. In our overscheduled lives, time spent in nature may seem like a luxury we can ill-afford, a dispensable commodity easily replaced by virtual and electronic experiences.

It is our children who are the most vulnerable to what Richard Louv, chairman of the Children & Nature Network, refers to as *nature-deficit disorder.* In *Last Child in the Woods: Saving Our Children From Nature Deficit Disorder,* Louv writes, "Reducing that deficit—healing the broken bond between our young and nature—is in our self-interest, not only because aesthetics or justice demands it, but also because our mental, physical, and spiritual health depends upon it."

Although we have twice the life expectancy of our ancestors, the quality of our lives is increasingly impacted with chronic physical, emotional, mental, and spiritual health issues. Improving our quality of life is about realigning with nature by living more like our ancestors. The ancients lived largely out-of-doors where they received plenty of sunshine, fresh air, and access to clean water. Their diets consisted of raw, unprocessed foods—free of sugar and grains until 10,000 to 15,000 years ago. They were very physically active and rested, slept, and played in sync with the rhythms of nature. Their close-knit communal living was rich with creativity, music, rituals, and ceremonies that marked the transitions of life and the seasons of nature.

A growing body of research has validated what our ancestors innately knew—exposure to nature is vital to health and development. Research studies indicate time spent in nature is powerfully therapeutic—naturally increasing physical activity, reducing stress, muscle tension, and blood pressure, relieving depression, improving concentration, and leaving one with a sense of well-being. Nature experiences enhance intelligence, creativity, and sensory skills, and heighten awareness of our surroundings.

In my personal and professional experience, I have found this enhanced awareness that occurs with nature experiences leads to increased awareness of our physical, emotional, mental, and spiritual selves—awareness that is critical to the healing process. The energetic effect of time spent outdoors heightens intuition, facilitates the processing of emotions, and brings peace and clarity to our everyday lives.

You may recall from chapter 2 that the instantaneous communication seen in the coordinated movement of a flock of birds or a school of fish occurs through wave resonance. When we observe and spend time in nature, our frequencies also become coordinated and synchronized with our environment through wave resonance.

When I became housebound due to the issues of Jacob's early years, I would retreat to our backyard to garden or meditate during his naps. Lying under an oak tree, I surrendered, allowing my subtle body to merge with the ground beneath me. In those moments I could feel myself vibrating in sync with the energy of the tree, and any separation between me and my environment ceased to exist.

In nature, there is no judgment. In nature, there are no victims—predators and prey are simply doing the dance of life. In nature, life exists in the moment. And in nature, we become aware of who we really are and our connection to everyone and everything around us.

Necessities for Health

Through our examination of modern research, coupled with what we know of the ancient way of life, we have explored the healing effects of *being* in nature. Now let's look at how we can promote and restore health through *observing* nature. In particular, what plants and animals require:

- Oxygen
- Water
- Nutrients
- Sunlight

In addition to these four basic needs, the health requirements of animals include:

- Rest
- Play
- Movement
- Community

We share these needs with plants and animals, yet all too often lack these basic elements for health in our daily life. These are the *laws of nature*—the requirement for adequate oxygen, water, and nutrients through "everyday energy medicine"; proper breathing, drinking, and eating; as well as sunlight, rest, play, movement, and nurturing contact with others. When our lives lack these basics—in effect *violating* natural laws—our health suffers. Living out of alignment with our innate, natural selves is incompatible with health.

In addition to these eight basic plant and animal needs, humans also benefit from:

- Creative Expression
- Sound and Music
- Ritual and Ceremony

These later categories may not seem necessary for health. We can certainly survive without creative expression, sound and music, or ritual and ceremony in our lives. However, a life without these elements is just that—merely surviving. A healing way of life with growth and transformation includes these powerful tools for health and healing.

It is important to note that, although these practices are entirely natural, in our modern lives we have strayed so far from living in sync with nature that integrating these natural health measures into our lives can paradoxically feel *unnatural*. At first, living a healing way of life may seem like a lot of hard work, especially when doing so causes a healing crisis or other unpleasant, though temporary, aspect of the healing process. The toxic effects of living against the laws of nature may require a "house cleaning" from a healing crisis before we can begin to experience the simple *pleasure* that comes from everyday energy medicine practices. In this brief survey of health needs and the natural practices that fulfill them, I think you will see how these measures can be easily woven into your everyday life, leading to health, happiness, and joy.

Oxygen

Oxygen is the most essential of all health requirements. We can survive without water for days and without food for months. But without oxygen, survival is in terms of minutes.

However, there is much more to breathing than survival and the exchange of oxygen and carbon dioxide. The act of breathing involves movement of structures within both the physical and subtle body—muscles, fascia, bones, organs, fluids, and the flow of energy. In spiritual traditions around the world, the word *breath* is synonymous with life force energy considered vital to healing. Breathing supplies every cell in the body with essential energy and is the most basic of all healing activities.

As a healing activity, conscious breathing and relaxation

techniques can relieve stress, anxiety, pain, muscle tension, insomnia, and inflammation. Conscious breathing improves immune function, increases circulation of blood and lymphatic fluid, activates the stress-relieving parasympathetic nervous system, speeds healing on all levels, and creates integration.

In addition to being a healing activity, how we breathe can become a healing *response*. Simply put, when your breathing becomes restricted from physical, emotional, mental, or spiritual distress, a *resistant* response—an energy disruption is present. Conversely, when you breathe slowly and deeply in response to distress, a *healing* response—the distress will move along with the flow of energy. However, the ability to choose a healing response to distress requires awareness.

Healing Breath

Breathing as a healing therapy can best be understood in terms of the steps of the healing process—awareness, compassion, trust, and surrender. Let's begin with awareness, particularly awareness of body tension. Take a moment to observe your body and your breathing, noticing where you may be restricted. I ask that you do this with compassion. Is your body relaxed? Is your breathing slow, smooth, and deep? Or is your body tense and your breathing fast or forceful? Although a hard body with a flat belly is desirable in our culture, a relaxed, supple body is required for natural, healthy breathing. By becoming conscious of your body tension, you gain access to the fear, grief, anger, or beliefs that are restricting your breathing.

In my work I have observed the increase in energy flow through the core nadis and chakra system of my clients that happens when I guide them in breathing consciously. Breathing can also increase energy flow to a particular area of the body, such as with the focused breathing technique I used earlier in this book while working with Katie and Steven. By intentionally "breathing into" areas that are tense or painful, the tissues, organs, fluids, and bone in that area become energetically activated, and we gain access to healing whatever suppressed emotion and disruption in energy was causing the tension and discomfort. An exercise in conscious and focused breathing can be found in the appendix.

Practicing breath-focused exercises increases awareness of beliefs, emotions, and level of resistance, as the way we breathe is a mirror of how we approach life. In *Free Your Breath, Free Your Life: How Conscious Breathing Can Relieve Stress, Increase Vitality, and Help You Live More Fully*, healing practitioner Dennis Lewis writes, "The process of health, healing and self-transformation is really about—the inner space and freedom to explore, to be, and to appreciate who or what I already am in my essence. The way we breathe, the way we participate day-by-day in the breath of life—the boundless life force that animates and connects us all—can play a vital role in this intimate exploration."

Breath is the link between the body, mind, and spirit; between the conscious and unconscious mind; between the upper and lower parts of the physical body; and between the upper and lower energy centers of the subtle body. Through conscious breathing, we can become aware of our entire being. Practicing full breathing allows us to take in more of life—living "larger," from our full potential, our higher selves.

As soon as we focus compassionately on the most fundamental of all bodily activities, *breathing*, we are instantly in the present moment and can begin to orient to who we really are—beings of energy. When we focus on breathing in a way that is slow, deep, expansive, and freeing, we become centered and have access to our deeper selves. This *centeredness* is the experience of being oriented to your core energy flow, your core being.

When we breathe in a restricted, superficial fashion, we are unconsciously suppressing our emotions and our core selves. While free, unrestricted breathing supports the healing process and is reflective of living from our higher self, restricted, inhibited breathing is associated with living from the limited "ego," or lower self.

In chapter 9, we explored Whitney's story—particularly how guilt had caused her to restrict her breathing and suppress her grief and disappointment over her unborn child's gender. The suppression had caused an energy disruption that resulted in bronchitis. But more to the point, in suppressing her natural emotion, Whitney was not living her truth, or from her core self.

Audrey also had issues with restricted breathing when experiencing guilt after her second miscarriage. Her inability to take in a deep breath interfered with her grief process and reflected an energy disruption that produced depression, anxiety, lower back tightness, and lack of creativity.

When I ask people to take a deep breath, they often do so forcefully. However, deep breathing exercises are about *allowing* breathing to happen smoothly and naturally, not about pushing all the air out of our lungs with exhalation, or forcing our lungs to expand wider to take in more air during inhalation. The level of restriction you observe in your breathing correlates to your level of resistance and suppression at any given moment—and that resistance and suppression cannot be released through force. Rather, resistance and suppression are released by allowing the expression of breathing restrictions while regarding them in a compassionate way. This creates trust, which facilitates surrender.

As an energy medicine therapist, focused observation of my client's breathing patterns during a session provides me with vital information on where they are in the healing process. When I observe a client spontaneously take a deep breath and slowly exhale with a sigh, followed by visible relaxation, it tells me they have just surrendered. This response indicates they have let go of attachment, ego-identification, fear, and the familiarity of their restricted state to embrace the unknown of a limitless, unrestricted state. But on a fundamental level, it tells me that an energy disturbance has just been released.

In feeling compassion for her irritated lungs, Whitney began to trust, and through that trust reached a state of surrender. In letting go, the energy disturbance that had caused her bronchitis released, and she was healed.

After Audrey experienced a healing release of guilt, her depression and anxiety started to improve. She decided to discontinue the medications she had been taking for anxiety and depression since her second pregnancy loss, as they made her feel sluggish and dull, and begin a program of daily conscious deep breathing techniques. With each deep breathing session, Audrey's anxiety lessened and her mood lifted. She experienced a deep sense of peace and a renewed passion for life. Her creativity returned with fresh, new ideas for her interior design business. "I didn't just get my old life back. I got a new and improved life," Audrey said.

Whatever you are feeling physically, emotionally, mentally, or spiritually—remember to keep breathing. Breath is the master key to health and healing, and as such, vital to any program of healing. Consistent daily practice of deep breathing helps us to tune in to our bodies and release stress before it builds up.

Breathing techniques that cultivate presence are not just applicable for childbirth—they are breathing for life!

Water Healing

Water healing, or hydrotherapy, is a method of healing as old as humanity. Modern hydrotherapy practices originated in the work of Vincent Priessnitz, a nineteenth century European healer. Priessnitz developed his water healing techniques after observing a wild deer heal its injured leg by submerging the limb in a cold mountain spring each day. Later, after being critically injured in a horse-drawn carriage accident, he fully recovered using applications of cold water bandages and drinking large amounts of water. Priessnitz was followed by many other natural health pioneers who are on record for being highly successful in treating acute and chronic health conditions with water healing.

Like other methods of healing, hydrotherapy restores energy flow to help the body heal itself. Both internal and external applications of water have health benefits and provide support during a healing crisis. In *The Complete Book of Water Healing: Using Earth's Most Essential Resource to Cure Illness, Promote Health, and Soothe and Restore Body, Mind, and Spirit,* herbalist Dian Dincin Buchman, Ph.D. writes, "But because we normally drink water only to quench thirst and as a solvent for our food, we tend to ignore its manifold health benefits and the fact that water is needed internally by every functioning cell and organ."

For proper body functioning, eight to twelve eight-ounce glasses of clean, filtered water per day are recommended. Pale, straw-colored urine is an indication that you are drinking an adequate amount of water. Water consumption decreases appetite, increases fat metabolism, relieves constipation, and can be used as a pick-me-up whenever one is feeling sluggish or sick. In the morning, drinking two to four cups of water at least 30 minutes before breakfast is the equivalent of taking an "internal shower," waking us up and initiating bodily processes.

Most people are aware of the relaxing benefits of external applications of warm and hot water. Hot water relieves aches and pains and creates perspiration, especially a steam bath, which assists the body in releasing wastes and toxins through the skin. However, a long hot bath can deplete energy and increase inflammation. Brief, regular exposure of the body to *cold* water is restorative, energizing, and strengthening. Cold water techniques mobilize the immune system and help build resistance to disease.

A cold compress covered with a dry cloth quickly becomes warm and is an effective self-care tool for a variety of health issues, such as fever, muscle and joint aches, hot flashes, and anxiety, or at the first sign of the flu or a cold An ice pack can relieve both acute and chronic congestion. Exposing either the whole body or the affected body part to alternating hot and cold water for fifteen seconds to three minutes each, ending with cold, increases circulation and decreases inflammation.

In addition to the energy healing techniques that helped Tess release her angry, critical, and hateful thoughts, she used cold compresses for chronic inflammation that developed after using anti-inflammatory medications. "I can feel a tingling sensation in my knee each time I put the cold compress on," she related. "The tingling starts in the knee and then I can feel it move down the lower leg until it reaches the bottom of my foot. Then my whole leg will start to feel warm." Through the use of water healing, Tess's inflammatory process was now resolving in alignment with Hering's third law of cure, from higher in the body to lower.

Tess noted that with this daily cold compress treatment, the inflammation in her knee alternately decreased and then slightly increased, with the length of pain-free time steadily rising. This back-and-forth meandering pattern and rising baseline pattern is inherent to the healing process. After a few weeks, the pain that had plagued Tess for months was gone.

A daily, brief barefoot walk through grass wet with morning dew is a powerful way to connect with nature, and an invigorating way to start your day. When this is not possible, a morning march in place in a tub with a few inches of cold water is also effective in strengthening the body and building vitality.

Of the myriad water healing techniques that can be found in Buchman's *The Complete Book of Water Healing,* I have found salt baths to be an excellent way to clear the energy field of any toxic energy that may have accumulated from daily stressors. Adding bath salts to bath water produces buoyancy, releases tension, and increases circulation.

As a medium for healing, water is unsurpassed. When we are immersed in water, especially without clothing, we are less inhibited, nearly weightless, and gently supported—reminiscent of our "water womb" origins. The primal state induced by water enhances presence, body-mind awareness, and emotional release. The limitless and freeing aspects of water make it an excellent environment for engaging in everyday energy medicine therapies, such as deep breathing, movement, vocalizations, and play.

Nutrients

Similar to the way we breathe, the way we approach eating is a mirror of our self-concepts and beliefs. According to nutritionist Deanna Minich, Ph.D., in *Chakra Foods for Optimal Health:*

A Guide to the Foods that can Improve Your Energy, Inspire Creative Changes, Open Your Heart, and Heal Body, Mind, and Spirit, "When we pay attention to what our body requires and view foods as healing entities, we get right to the heart of why we have manifested chronic diseases or eating dysfunctions."

That "paying attention" begins with observing your eating habits without judgment or criticism. Do you eat in response to emotional distress? Or do you forget to eat because slowing down and taking the time to nourish yourself might allow what you are avoiding in the darkness to come to the surface? Do you deny yourself food when you are hungry, or do you overfeed yourself? Do you nurture yourself with nourishing food, or do you abuse yourself with junk food?

Once aware of your eating patterns, you have a choice to respond to any dysfunctional behavior in an accepting, trust-building way, or with self-rejection, which perpetuates the energetic disruption causing the eating issue. As we have learned, the impulse to soothe inner wounds with food is a powerful one. You cannot "overpower" this impetus to numb painful emotions. The World Health Organization identifies obesity as a worldwide epidemic, but the path to achieving optimal weight is not through deprivation or "will power," or by substituting processed foods with artificial fats and artificial sweeteners for "real" food.

A vital component of self-love is nourishing yourself with high-quality, high-*vibrational* foods that are compatible with your energy systems. But how do you determine which foods are in your best interest? There are several methods for doing so, but first let's look at research on food vibrational levels in general.

Through Kirlian photography and dowsing methods, researchers have determined that while food that has been frozen or dehydrated retains its vitality, canned and processed foods have little to no energetic frequency. Processed cow's milk, juices, and baby formula are essentially "dead" food, as are cooked meats, coffee, tea, chocolate, white bread, white flour, white sugar, margarine, jams, and alcohol. These processed foods are a drain on body resources, as they lack the energy required to digest them. The digestive enzymes inherent to raw foods are destroyed during processing methods such as canning and pasteurization. In addition, when foods are processed with heat, particularly fats and proteins, toxins are created, including free radicals—unstable organic molecules that damage body tissues and contribute to aging.

Unprocessed foods, such as raw fruits and vegetables, sprouted seeds, and raw cow's milk and human milk, are "alive" in that their nutritional components and enzymatic activity are intact. They contain antioxidants that destroy free radicals and have a high vibrational frequency. This vibrational frequency produces a healing physiological response in the body—maintaining proper body pH and promoting detoxification.

Although we have established that raw foods have high vibrational frequencies, no single eating plan is going to be right for everyone. *Dr. Mercola's Total Health Cookbook and Program,* by natural health expert Joseph Mercola, M.D., includes a paper-and-pencil test for determining one's metabolic type, along with an eating program and recipes for each of his metabolic types. Dr. Mercola's program also advocates the use of EFT (Emotional Freedom Techniques) for removing energy blocks to improving eating habits. Another paper and pencil questionnaire found in Dr. Minich's *Chakra Foods for Optimal Health* can determine energy center issues and which foods can correct those imbalances.

You can also determine which foods are right for you by

observing how you feel after you eat. When a food is energy-disrupting, the effects on your personal physiology can create any number of physical, emotional, mental, and spiritual symptoms, including restricted breathing and muscle weakness. Individuals with a high level of body awareness may notice these subtle symptoms that occur when certain foods disrupt their energy systems. As my awareness increased through the healing process, I noticed how my legs felt wobbly with weakness when certain foods and drinks even touched my lips. I also observed sensations of slight nausea and fatigue. If you are not aware of these symptoms, testing muscle strength can pinpoint which foods are energy-disrupting.

Muscle testing, or kinesiology, is the most common method to "ask your body" whether a food is right for you. Instructions for muscle testing can be found on the Internet, or in *The Ultimate Healing System: The Illustrated Guide to Muscle Testing & Nutrition*, by nutritional research pioneer Donald Lepore, N.D. You can also create your own method of measuring muscle strength. As the artificial sweetener aspartame is universally energy-disrupting, it can be used as a "control" in muscle testing.

A common type of muscle testing involves bringing the tips of the thumb and little finger of your non-dominant hand together to form a circle, and then inserting the thumb and index finger of the dominant hand inside that circle. Using the same amount of pressure to maintain the circle with your non-dominant fingers as you use to break the circle with your dominant fingers will determine muscle strength. If the circle does not break in the presence of a food substance, the food is compatible with your energy systems. If the circle created by your fingers breaks from muscle weakness, the food is disruptive to your energy systems.

Muscle testing can also be used for detecting negative belief systems. For example, if I am unable to maintain muscle strength while making a statement such as "I am a worthy person," I know that to my energy systems this statement is a "lie." The consciousness states associated with negative belief systems—shame, guilt, apathy, grief, fear, desire, anger, and pride—produce energy flow disruption which results in muscle weakness. The consciousness states of courage, neutrality, willingness, acceptance, unconditional love, peace, and grace are associated with energy flow and physical strength.

Using high vibrational foods that are compatible with our energy systems as energy medicine has a detoxifying effect. This effect works on all levels—physical, emotional, mental, spiritual, and energetic. I'd like to give you an example of this action in Jim, the gentleman I worked with whose mother abandoned him when he was a child. Jim originally sought my help for healing from asthma.

When I first met Jim, it was clear to me that he carried unexpressed grief related to the loss of his mother's presence in his life from childhood, although he was unaware of this. Our work together had only been partially successful in tapping into that deeply repressed grief. As we discussed everyday energy medicine practices he could use on his own, Jim was intuitively guided to focus on detoxifying raw foods. His intention for the nutritional program he chose was to improve his physical health and asthma. But in the healing crisis that ensued, unexpected and powerful feelings of abandonment, grief, and loss suddenly surfaced, as if his mother had left his life yesterday, not twenty years ago. Through the use of food as energy medicine, Jim's repressed emotions were at last fully available for expression, and through acceptance of that expression his asthma did improve.

Sunlight

Another detoxifying energy medicine practice involves the use of *sunlight*. We've all seen pet cats and dogs pick the sunniest spots in our homes to lie in the sun. They instinctively know what people have known for eons; sunlight is vital for restoring and maintaining good health.

Historically, sunlight therapy, or heliotherapy, has been effectively used in the prevention of tetanus and gangrene in war wounds, as well as the treatment of tuberculosis, smallpox, and other serious health conditions. However, with the discovery of antibiotics, the use of therapeutic sunlight to treat infectious diseases no longer seemed necessary. Sunlight therapy fell further out of favor with the discovery of a "hole" in the ozone layer, coupled with increasing numbers of skin cancers and cataracts. As such, current guidelines recommend severely limiting sun exposure and protecting the skin with broad spectrum sunscreens. We now live our lives almost entirely indoors in buildings that are no longer designed to maximize sunlight. Unfortunately, indoor living lifestyles and avoiding sunlight have serious health consequences.

The truth is there is no evidence that depletion of the ozone layer has caused an increased incidence of skin cancer. Nor is there any evidence that avoiding sunlight, using sunscreen, or wearing sunglasses prevents skin cancer or cataracts. Although damage to the skin from sunburn or other trauma *does* increase the risk of skin cancer, a far greater risk to health has been attributed to a *lack* of sunlight, as well as a diet deficient in antioxidants and exposure of the skin to toxic chemicals from products such as cosmetics and many sunscreens.

In *The Healing Sun: Sunlight and Health in the 21st Century,* complementary medicine practitioner Richard Hobday, Ph.D. writes "Sunlight may cause skin cancer but, paradoxically, there is growing scientific evidence that the sun's rays could play a key role in preventing and ameliorating a number of serious degenerative and infectious diseases." I have no doubt that shunning the sun during my teens, coupled with overexposure in college, were key factors in developing malignant melanoma. This potentially fatal form of skin cancer could have been avoided through safe and proper sun exposure.

Healing With Sun Energy

Sunlight has long been used as a therapy to prevent and cure disease, although until recently the mechanism of action was unknown. Today we know that heliotherapy uses energy from the sun in the form of electromagnetic waves. This sunlight energy is vital for the healthy functioning of systems throughout the body. These waves of ultraviolet radiation irradiate blood in capillaries near the surface of the skin, increasing the formation of white blood cells called lymphocytes that are necessary for a healthy immune system. This energetic action also increases the oxygen content of the blood and accelerates elimination of toxic chemicals from the body. For example, when the skin of infants who are jaundiced is exposed to sunlight, the excessive bilirubin in the blood that is causing the jaundice is broken down, and the color of the infant's skin returns to normal.

Not only does sunlight energy detoxify and strengthen the immune system, it also synthesizes vitamin D production in the skin, essential for healthy teeth and bones and in prevention of the serious diseases and cancers associated with vitamin D deficiency.

Such a deficiency is linked with depressive illnesses such as Seasonal Affect Disorder (SAD); cancer of the skin, breast, colon, ovaries, and prostate; diabetes, high blood pressure, heart disease, multiple sclerosis, psoriasis, rickets, osteoporosis, and tuberculosis. Heliotherapy can prevent and treat these disease conditions due to the ability of sunlight to: lower blood cholesterol, blood sugar, and blood pressure levels; regulate hormonal processes; balance our internal biological rhythms; and kill bacteria. In particular, it has become imperative to recover lost knowledge of sunlight's natural antibacterial effect, given the escalating issue of antibiotic-resistant bacterial infections.

Although vitamin D deficiency is widely recognized as a public health threat, the artificial solutions imposed in the West are inadequate and potentially dangerous. Substituting artificial light for natural sunlight energy disrupts body physiology and production of melatonin, a neurohormone that regulates the wake-sleep cycle. In addition, studies have linked fluorescent lighting with malignant melanoma. The use of vitamin D supplements, as well as the widespread practice of fortifying the public food supply with vitamin D, are unreliable and carry a risk of toxicity. Given that both sun avoidance and sunburns have health consequences and artificial substitutes are unsatisfactory, how can we maintain healthy vitamin D levels when there is no sunlight, and safely do so when there is?

The key to safely receiving the benefits of sunbathing is through brief, regular, and gradually increasing sun exposure. Such practices prevent sunburn by properly preparing the skin. It is especially important for individuals with pale skin to follow these guidelines, as research indicates that it is only among the fair-skinned segment of the population that the incidence of malignant melanoma is increasing. That increase is attributed to sun avoidance, which leaves the skin ill-prepared for exposure and contributes to burning.

Claire decided to try heliotherapy to heal any deficiencies in her immune system function that contributed to her frequent infections. Following guidelines for optimal vitamin D production, Claire began daily sunbathing without sunscreen in the cooler temperatures of early spring mornings, continuing into the early summer. As a fair-skinned individual, she began with five minutes of sun exposure to her feet and ankles. Those with darker skin can begin with longer exposure. Claire gradually increased the length of time and amount of skin she exposed to include the full leg, exposing the torso last, while wearing a hat to protect her sensitive facial, neck, and upper chest skin.

In a few weeks, Claire had worked up to a half-hour of sunbathing. By using the guidelines established by pioneers of heliotherapy, which can be found in Hobday's *The Healing Sun: Sunlight and Health in the 21st Century*, her body could synthesize and store enough vitamin D in body fat and skeletal muscle to maintain levels during low-light winter months, while avoiding a skin-damaging sunburn.

Claire was delighted to share with me that the chronic infections that plagued her had vanished and her energy level was much improved, an effect that was still evident through the winter that followed.

Sleep

Another consequence of our lost connection to nature through living our lives almost entirely indoors is the effect on our *sleep*. Our attempts to control nature by replacing natural sunlight energy with artificial sources of energy have produced epidemic levels of sleep disorders. Excessive artificial light in our indoor and outdoor environments, avoidance of the sun during the day, as well as the use of artificial sedatives to sleep and artificial stimulants to wake up, have proved disastrous to health.

According to the National Sleep Foundation, 75 percent of Americans *voluntarily* cut their sleep short. We are averaging two fewer hours of sleep a night than our ancestors did only a hundred years ago, and the incidence of insomnia is steadily rising. We simply aren't getting enough sleep, and the sleep we do get is poor in quality. In essence, we are in a state of *resisting* the night—but why?

According to psychologist Rubin R. Naiman, Ph.D., our rejection of night is an extension of rejecting ourselves. In *The Healing Night: The Science and Spirit of Sleeping, Dreaming, and Awakening,* Naiman writes, "Our disturbed relationship with night is ultimately rooted in our discomfort with and denial of the dark side of our own selves." When we reject parts of ourselves and relegate them to the darkness of the shadow, the resulting energy disturbance has a direct impact on our sleep. We unconsciously avoid sleep and deny our need for rest because slowing down can allow what is suppressed to surface.

The consequences to our health from this resistance to night are great. When we avoid darkness by extending the day with artificial light, melatonin production is inhibited. Melatonin is the hormone produced by the pineal gland that regulates the sleep-wake cycle, controls reproductive hormones, and strengthens the immune system. Sleep disorders and inadequate sleep disturb our energetic rhythms and are associated with chronic fatigue syndrome, fibromyalgia, heart disease, stroke, inflammation, obesity, premature aging, diabetes, and mental health and memory issues.

But just as damaging to our health as sleep loss is *dream loss,* which has been linked to depression and cancer. Dream loss represents a loss of one's "inner life," a disconnection from our core energy flow and spiritual selves.

While sleep deprivation causes sleepiness, dream deprivation results in difficulties with concentration, perceptual distortions, and fatigue. We cope with these issues by using alcohol and sleeping pills to fall asleep at night, and caffeine, sugar, personal drama and electronic stimulation to stay awake during the day. Unfortunately, the use of alcohol and medications such as sleeping pills and anti-depressants only worsens the situation by suppressing melatonin production, which disrupts sleep and suppresses dreaming.

Healing the Night

Healing our relationship to night is about becoming aware of our need to rest, engaging in practices that restore our natural rhythms, and reconnecting with our core essence through dream and shadow work.

In our hyperproductive culture, we tend to deny our need for rest. This denial suppresses our natural cycles, in effect *flattening* our rhythms. In this state we are never completely at rest at night and never fully conscious during the day. Although we label rest as being lazy and suppress it, it is as important to our health as exercise.

Scientists have discovered that we require about twenty minutes of restful activity out of every ninety minutes of our day. When you notice yourself feeling distracted and tired during the day, it's a signal to briefly stop whatever activity you are engaged in and allow yourself some time for stretching, deep breathing, meditation, or a nap, until your energy level returns. Honoring your need for rest also creates space for dreams—both during the day and at night.

Restoring natural rhythms includes practices that respect vital transitions that occur from day to night, and night to day. In the evening, the transition to sleep can be eased by decreasing activity, dimming lights, and avoiding consumption of alcohol and caffeine. Mornings are an opportunity to transition from unconscious to conscious and celebrate a new day. This is best accomplished through gradual awakening, rather than being startled awake, and establishing the sun as an energy source through exposure to refreshing morning sunlight. Morning and evening rituals and spiritual practices, such as prayer, meditation, affirmations, and journaling, help us to set intentions for and embrace the day, and let go of the day's angst and surrender to the night. These transition times of day and night are also opportunities for increasing one's state of consciousness and gaining insights through the recording of dreams.

Dream and Shadow Work

In the West, dreams have been largely devalued, minimized, and feared. But working with our dreams provides us access to deep healing through the treasure trove of unconscious information and suppressed emotions that both night dreams and daydreams contain. Although daydreams are typically viewed as a waste of time, research indicates that both types of dreams activate problem-solving areas of the brain and are a time when the brain integrates learning. The challenges we face to tapping into this source of healing are the fear of looking at what we have suppressed, simply remembering dreams, and finally, being able to understand them.

Remembering dreams begins with setting the intention to do so upon retiring, keeping a journal near the bed, and taking the time to record them upon waking. Before I began a healing way of life, I rarely remembered my dreams. Yet, as soon as I made the decision to remember, I was able to do this. Considering dream content in a relaxed, detached state of mind, free of criticism, creates the opening for the dream's message to be revealed. Sometimes the meaning of a dream does not become clear for some time, even years. By recording dream images and any parallels between dream material and daytime occurrences in a journal, we can begin to identify symbolic meanings, patterns, and recurrent themes for later reference when more information becomes available. Recurrent dreams will often continue until we grasp the meaning.

Although dreams contain some symbols that are universal, it is more valuable to consider what each element of a dream *personally* represents. For example, child characters that appear in a dream are commonly associated with the "inner child"—that part of our psyche thought to contain childhood experiences and emotions. But for a deeper interpretation, consider what you personally associate with the specific characteristics of your dream characters, as well as the context in which they appear in your dreams.

Rita had recurring nightmares of a wild-eyed, angry woman with black hair who was trying to break into her home. In the dreams, Rita was terrified and barricaded the door to keep the woman out. When the color black appears in our dreams, in this case the color of the woman's hair, it is typically associated with shadow material. Similarly, the color black is associated with absence of energy flow. When we repress aspects of ourselves into the shadow, we disturb the flow of energy through our energy systems. By working with our dreams, we have an opportunity to discover what we have disowned and suppressed in the shadow and bring it to consciousness, thereby restoring energy flow and creating wholeness and health.

In considering the black-haired woman in the dream as a representation of a disowned aspect of herself, Rita began to view her nightmares with a new perspective. While imagining what the dream character might be trying to tell her, she recognized how "barricading the door" against the woman in the dream was a symbol of her resistance to her own anger. By metaphorically "opening the door," Rita was able to connect with her disowned fury at not being accepted as a child—the rage that the dream character expressed. In time, Rita saw this disowned part of herself as her ally, a barometer for inauthenticity that indicated when she was not being true to herself and her emotions.

When she made peace with the black-haired woman of her dreams, Rita's nightmares stopped, her anxiety and insomnia lessened, and her Graves' disease stabilized. By becoming aware of what she had rejected, and then embracing all parts of herself, including her anger, Rita was able to heal her relationship with the night and her fear of her darkness.

As our spiritual awareness increases through dream work, we can actually become aware that we are dreaming *while* we are dreaming. This is referred to as *lucid* dreaming. During a lucid dream, you can ask the characters in the dream questions about the meaning of the dream. What better way to obtain information than directly from the source! Working with our night dreams, daydreams, and lucid dreams can provide guidance through the healing process, furnishing valuable feedback on where we are in that process.

Play

Like dreams, another important element for health that has been largely devalued is *play*. Although play may seem a guilty pleasure that wastes precious time and serves no purpose, research indicates otherwise. In *Play: How it Shapes the Brain, Opens the Imagination, and Invigorates the Soul,* psychiatrist, clinical researcher, and play behavior expert Dr. Stuart Brown writes, "... the opposite of play is not work—the opposite of play is depression." Similar to nature, sleep, and dream deficits, a deficit in play produces pessimism and robs our lives of pleasure.

We can best understand the importance of play by looking at research on animal play. Play has been observed throughout the animal kingdom—even in ants, fish and octopi. Although play does not appear to be a survival-based behavior for animals, nor has it been attributed to skills practice, the fact that animals do engage in play speaks to its importance. In his study of grizzly bear behavior, renowned animal play expert Bob Fagen discovered that bears who were the best at survival and had the largest brains were the ones who *played the most.* Why? Because it is through play that animals and humans alike try out different scenarios and novel experiences, rehearsing for life's challenges and unpredictability. Researchers from the fields of neuroscience, developmental biology, and psychology are in agreement that play is a biological impetus, is key to adaptation and survival, and stimulates neural growth and shapes the brain.

So what exactly is play? Although play is the basis of art, fashion, movies, books, games, and sports, it is not organized, rigid, or competitive. By its nature, play is purposeless, voluntary, uninhibited, improvisational, varied, pleasurable, and *energizing*. Play is also preconscious, preverbal, and *primal*. When engaged in play, we lose our sense of time. More to the point, play is a state of mind that just plain makes us feel *good*.

The benefits of play are many and varied—from strengthening social relationships to fostering compassion and creativity. Through play our burdens are eased, optimism is renewed, and we open up to new possibilities. Play adds excitement and adventure to our lives that ripples out through everything we do, increasing productivity and happiness. Corporate America is beginning to recognize the importance of play through the hiring of individuals with a strong play history. Why? Because they recognize that innovation comes through play and those lacking in childhood play are also lacking in problem-solving skills.

Although play is clearly good for us, cultural factors can prevent us from playing. Earlier we discussed the emphasis of early independence in our culture. This, coupled with the belief that the need for play is restricted to childhood, can cause us to suppress both our need for play and the child part of us. While it is important to reach maturity, this is achieved through taking responsibility for our actions, not by disconnecting from our lifelong need to play. When that need has become suppressed, it is through play that we can reconnect and integrate with the child self.

Healing does not have to be serious business. It's important to relax, laugh, and have fun through the process—doing so can mediate the effects of a healing crisis. Smiling is considered a universal play signal, an invitation for contact and connection, as is relaxed body posture, soft facial expressions, and "curvilinear" body movements. When we use play signals, we are reaching out energetically and connecting with others. But on a deeper level, such nonverbal invitations come from our authentic, core selves— our ultimate truth.

I learned about energy dynamics and explored the subtle body through *play*. My investigations and experiments with dowsing rods, a pendulum, and my inner senses were conducted with an attitude of playfulness. And my ongoing education in the energetic effects of play has come through observing my own energy and those of clients.

When I am engaged in play, my body vibrates and buzzes all over. And a playful attitude introduced in a healing session acts as a catalyst, accelerating the release of disruptions in energy systems and producing a sense of lightness. However, when suggesting that clients use their imagination in a playful way, at first they may be resistant. Although play is how we learn, all too often we are so afraid of making a mistake that we shut down the flow of energy.

Through our work together, some of my clients, such as Deidra, have regained childhood memories of playing with energy. Deidra recalled observing the movement of energy around people, animals, and plants, and playing with the balloon-like sensation that energy produced between her hands. If these natural explorations didn't occur in your childhood, or you have no recollection of such, it's never too late.

Mandy clearly remembered playing with energy as a child, and drawing pictures of her family members with their energy systems. But as she grew up, she dismissed these experiences as her imagination, not realizing that imagination is how we access our intuition. During her achievement-focused high school years, and again as a young adult weighed down by financial and career concerns, she had lost touch with the playful child part of her.

When I suggested Mandy incorporate play in her healing program, she began taking out her sketch pad on a daily basis, approaching the activity in a playful manner. Mandy reported that, as she doodled on the paper, the stress of the day would melt away, lightening her mood and bringing pleasure to her life.

After Deidra regained her childhood memory of playing with energy, I asked her, "What other ways did she enjoy playing when you were a kid?" She instantly became more animated as she talked about exploring the racks of books at the library, an activity she had recently resumed. Deidra also recalled how much she enjoyed skipping, swinging on a swing, and dancing around the house as a child. "It sounds like you relished playful movement as a child. Is there a way you can recapture some of that now?" I asked her.

After our discussion, Deidra began injecting a playful attitude in her life, putting a spring in her step even if she was just doing housework and even if she felt sluggish or stiff. She was surprised to find that this simple change in attitude lessened her pain, decreased her tension, and increased her energy.

When we are judging and critical of ourselves, it can be difficult to be uninhibited and playful about learning. The use of exploratory movement can help us get past our fears and defenses that interfere with play, allowing access to our deeper, primal self. So give yourself permission to make a mistake, try out different scenarios, move, and *play*.

Movement

When we move and exercise, we aren't just moving our physical bodies. We are also creating movement in our subtle bodies, raising our vibrational level and balancing our energetic and

biological rhythms. As such, movement has a powerfully positive effect on our health. Natural health expert Joseph Mercola,
M.D. advises the public to think of exercise as a *drug*—a potent
drug, free of side effects, that has the potential to cure serious
diseases such as diabetes. Indeed, research indicates exercise can
be more effective in treating depression than medication, and can
be an excellent treatment for insomnia, weight issues, and insulin
resistance.

Although organized exercise programs that utilize equipment,
classes, or personal training are beneficial to health, they are not
necessarily *healing*. You may recall that healing is a continuum,
and that staying at any point on that continuum is stagnation. The
repetitive movements that characterize many exercise programs
can reinforce held patterns in our lives that arise from trauma,
thereby creating stagnation. *Healing* movements are spontaneous,
creative, intuitive, and playful.

Healing through movement includes the use of energy medicine movement modalities. These movement arts evolved from
self-defense and spiritual practices in the East, and from dance
in the West. Eastern movement arts, such as yoga, T'ai Chi, and
martial arts, emphasize *being* rather than *doing*—a meditative
state of mind that requires one to be in the moment. Practicing
Eastern movement arts can enhance personal growth by height-
ening intuition, increasing awareness of energetic movement,
building "inner" strength, and balancing energetic flow.

Western movement arts, such as Pilates and Continuum, are
educational in nature, increasing body awareness and helping
us break free from habitual and limited movement and thinking
patterns. While children are naturally explorative, spontaneous,
and playful with their movements, adults tend to become fixed

and rigid in how they move and think. This rigidity arises from the cumulative effect of life's traumas and the need to avoid the anxiety that can arise when we venture outside our comfort zone. Movement arts also help to fill in any gaps in our development and restore energetic flow throughout our energy systems.

When Steven fell off his bicycle as a child and never rode again, he lost confidence in his body and began limiting participation in other childhood movement activities. And although the traumatic effects of his fiancée's death were released through energy healing therapies, Steven's life was still being unduly influenced by this earlier event. Neither falling off a bicycle nor failing to learn how to ride one is inherently traumatic. Learning to ride a bike is also not necessary for an individual's development. However, with Steven, the bicycle incident created a pattern of limitation that globalized to all aspects of his life. Even after his addictions and health issues resolved, making it possible for him to return to collegiate teaching, he still felt limited in his career and relationships, reluctant to try anything new and unable to follow through with creative ideas.

With some encouragement, Steven began to explore movement arts. Given that he never learned how to balance himself on a bicycle, he decided to try yoga, which features poses that improve core strength and balance. Steven was surprised to find that practicing yoga decreased his anxiety and stress, lowered his blood pressure, and increased his confidence in his body. Through yoga, Steven broke through limitations and gained confidence in his body-mind to try new things. Adding a movement art to his healing program served as a catalyst, accelerating his healing process.

Regardless of whether you choose a formal exercise program, a movement art, or decide to explore creative, intuitive movements with a movement therapist or on your own, movement is integral to a healing way of life. Additional information on healing movement and Eastern or Western movement arts can be found in Mirka Knaster's *Discovering the Body's Wisdom.*

Community

Thus far in our survey of health needs and the self-help healing practices that fulfill them, you may have gotten the impression that healing is a solitary pursuit. As it happens, close, intimate relationships are as vital to our health as any of the health needs explored in this chapter. Simply put, we *need* people—not just to mitigate stress and relieve isolation—but to learn from, to add meaning to our lives, and to provide the feedback necessary for growth and the formation of healthy self-concepts.

Earlier in this book, we talked about how lasting and increased happiness is associated with positive interactions and connections with others, especially when those connections are associated with acts of generosity and compassion. In studies of human happiness, participants considered close relationships the most essential factor to their well-being. In other research, social support was found to decrease anxiety and depression, and to dramatically increase survival rates from serious illnesses such as breast cancer and heart attacks. Likewise, social support has been proven to double the chance of conception for infertile women during a conventional treatment cycle. Of the dozens of women who attended the local infertility support group meetings I led for Resolve, the national infertility organization, the conception rate was similarly high for attendees, regardless of what type of treatment they were using, if any.

However, Newtonian-Cartesian influences that value

individuality over connectivity can prevent us from receiving the benefits of a social support network. The effect of this strong societal influence begins with the parent-child relationship and continues throughout life. When we don't get our dependency needs met in the first years of life, it creates strain in later relationships. And cultural emphasis on individualism can interfere with the development of social support that would take pressure off the few close relationships we have. The void left in this absence of social support is often filled with artificial stimulants, such as electronic media, and through over-scheduling our lives, creating a chronic state of busyness. These attempts to numb, suppress, and *decrease* the anxiety and loneliness of social isolation only serve to create *more* social isolation, and more anxiety and loneliness.

Psychotherapist Dr. Will Miller suggests that the erosion of close, personal relationships is directly responsible for the high rates of stress, divorce, depression, rudeness, road rage, and substance abuse that characterize modern life. In *Refrigerator Rights: Why we need to let people into our hearts, our homes (and our refrigerators)... and how to bring even more close relationships into our lives,* Dr. Miller writes, "Taking steps to repopulate my daily world with emotionally close relationships has been the single most effective force in reducing my stress levels." Given this, no therapy or medicine, whether biochemical or energetic in nature, can substitute for the depression-relieving and anxiety-reducing effects of strong social support. As such, the efforts and actions we take to maintain current relationships and build new ones *are* energy medicine.

It is clear that the presence of close relationships and strong social support in our lives is vital, but what specific actions create connection, and how do we find compatible people to connect with? According to Dr. Miller, "…our culture puts far too much emphasis on temperamental compatibility and lifestyle conformity as criteria for emotional closeness with others." In fact, it is through *diversity* that we grow—not some ideal of perfect compatibility.

Close relationships can be forged between individuals from all walks of life, and that closeness is created simply by spending time with others in ordinary, everyday activities, and being vulnerable enough to share our feelings. This sharing of ourselves coupled with shared experiences creates connection and intimacy in a deepening process that grows and nurtures relationships, creating the feeling of *belonging*—a hallmark of effective social support.

As the blockages in her energy systems cleared and Vanessa shifted to a prevailing state of higher frequency, enriching situations to connect to others began appearing in her life. In describing how she felt helping with a local Habitat for Humanity project, Vanessa replied, "I was practically on a "high" working alongside the other volunteers. We were all so different—different ages, backgrounds, life situations—yet I felt so connected to them. I've always tried to connect with people just like me, but that usually ended with disappointment and hurt. Now that I know what it feels like to belong, I want more of these experiences!"

There are a few caveats to consider in relationship-building as energy medicine. A healing way of life includes observing the energy dynamics underlying your relationships, specifically the nature of the frequencies that others are mirroring. As spiritual connections are at work in our relationships, whether we are conscious of it or not, the question to ask is this: What are the people in my life reflecting back to me? If you are in the frequency of loving and accepting yourself, you will attract more love and acceptance in your life. If you are experiencing hurt and rejection in your relationships, this provides valuable information about the state of your frequencies, beliefs, level of suppression, and energy blocks.

When we vibrate in frequencies such as unloved, unworthy, or unsafe, we can attract people who are toxic, violate our boundaries, and devalue us—people who make us feel bad and only take from us. We may think that's all we can get—that we don't deserve supportive, reciprocal relationships. In considering the nature of our relationships as a "mirror," we see that through awareness, all connections have the potential to be healing, even when hurtful and traumatic. However, that doesn't mean we have to continue those types of connections.

Although communities provide an environment for the shared experiences that grow a social support network, particularly faith-based communities, such groups and organizations should not require you to deny your truth in order to be accepted. If a relationship is characterized by the use of force and is outright devaluing or abusive—the path of action is clear. But usually we have to carefully weigh the pros and cons of dysfunctional individual or group relationships, and decide if there is anything further to be gained from connections that are dysfunctional, toxic, or draining.

Once we recognize the healing messages in our relationships, we can take back our projections and feel gratitude for what we have learned. But this does not mean we have to live with disrespect and devaluing of our shared feelings. We can choose to limit contact with those who devalue us, or move on altogether. Sometimes it is in our best interest to leave the relationship, the organization, the job, or the religion when the price of continuing, in terms of health and well-being, becomes too great.

As we have discussed, research indicates close, supportive relationships greatly benefit our health and well-being. But even ending a relationship can be healing, if the healing process that it initiates is allowed to fully express without suppression, and the death, transition and rebirth cycles that ensue are embraced. For many of my clients, difficult endings such as divorce, or leaving the religion they were raised in, have served as catalysts. These situations create an entry into a healing way of life, followed by a painful but fruitful transition process that ultimately creates *transformation.*

This concludes our survey of the basic health needs we humans share with plants and animals. Now let's examine our higher level needs for creativity, sound and music, and ritual.

Creativity

Regardless of what type of healing professional you may consult for your issues, you cannot rely solely on that assistance for healing. Healing does not just occur during the one-hour or so time frame of a healing appointment. I have found that clients who adopt healing as a way of life experience the greatest success in transforming their issues. By engaging in healing activities in our everyday lives, we take responsibility for our own healing process.

We have talked about the importance of fully expressing distressing thoughts and emotions in the process of healing. Creative endeavors such as art and writing provide an excellent medium for such expression. In *Healing through Writing: A Journaling Guide to Emotional and Spiritual Growth,* mental health therapist and social worker Anthony Parnell explores the use of writing as a powerful tool for healing.

Parnell gained insight into the ongoing nature of the healing process with the realization that, even after years of personal healing work, he was still not "done." With the revelation that childhood wounds he thought were resolved were still an issue, he writes, "… I slowly began to develop a more realistic expectation of my process of emotional and spiritual growth. I realized and began to accept that wholeness and balance are not fixed states of being. Rather, they are states of existence that constantly must be nurtured and maintained by exercising daily awareness." Through daily journaling, he found a medium for expression of his thoughts and emotions, becoming aware of his limiting negative beliefs, and experiencing transformation.

Daily journaling can become a tool for documenting how we are feeling each day, and a means to identify the different patterns at work in our healing process. Through the practice of journaling, we can become aware of the meandering pattern, spiral pattern, and Hering's Laws of Cure in our personal healing journey. By examining our daily writings, we are better able to identify when we are experiencing a healing crisis, or a death, transition, or rebirth cycle.

Healing through writing can be accomplished through poetry, daily narratives, and letters to self. In *Radical Forgiveness*, Colin Tipping suggests writing a series of letters to fully express victim consciousness, and then burning them as a powerful tool for healing. Other methods of healing through writing include the recording of dreams, synchronicities, significant events, inner questions, beliefs, and personal goals. Through this practice we can increase awareness, gain insights, find solutions, and reach acceptance.

After Brooke's dramatic energetic shift from dependence on others for approval to reconnection with the universal energy field, she began daily rituals of meditation, music, and journaling to strengthen her spiritual connection and core energy flow. Writing in her journal about her continuing struggle to set boundaries and say "no" to others helped Brooke clarify the motives behind her decision-making regarding time-management. With the focus that came from writing down her thoughts, Brooke was able to identify when she was responding from a need for approval versus from her intuition. Each time Brooke made a choice to align with her core and her truth, energy flow was restored and her autoimmune conditions began to reverse.

Expressing ourselves through art may be even more effective than using words. Research indicates that we experience our thoughts, feelings, and emotions first as images and then as words. According to expressive arts educator and certified holistic health counselor Barbara Ganim, "If emotions are held in the body-mind as images, then imagery rather than words would be the most direct route to get in touch with these painful emotions, and then to release the images of these feelings and emotions as art."

In *Art and Healing: Using Expressive Art to Heal Your Body, Mind, and Spirit,* Ganim examines healing emotional wounds through varied mediums of expression, including drawing, painting, sculpture, and collage. Art therapy does not require any artistic talent, and is one of the few modes of healing accepted in conventional medical settings, as the creation of art has been found to improve immune system dysfunction.

Healing through Creativity

After Sophie had weight loss surgery, followed by a

physician-recommended eating plan that included highly processed "diet food" with artificial sweeteners, she experienced a
health crisis precipitated by severe nutritional deficiencies. Earlier
in her life, she had painted beautiful inner images that she was
unable to express verbally. After her surgery, when her health
began to unravel and daily life became a struggle, she again turned
to art. Of her experience, Sophie related:

"As I started painting, I noticed that the whole world went
silent, and still. When I say that it went silent I mean there could
be chaos happening, but nothing bothered me. All I noticed was
my brushes, paint, and canvas. While painting, I was no longer
anxious or upset. My mind was clear and relaxed. It was as if I
was meditating. Painting whatever I felt allowed me to release
and experience myself, turning my feelings into art even when the
painting came from a dark place. I felt as though I was letting go
of those feelings with each stroke."

Through art, Sophie found a vehicle for expressing the
emotions that could no longer be suppressed through overeating, which was no longer an option with her new, smaller
stomach. Although the surgery had caused severe fatigue and
nutritional deficiencies, those complications became the catalyst to heal the deeper emotional wounds that had caused
her obesity in the first place. Sophie's experience using art
for healing led to a new career in professional photography.
Both writing and art provide a *safe* means of expressing emotions, which is especially valuable for those who have difficulty
verbalizing their emotions, or when words are simply inadequate.
Writing down or drawing our most private thoughts and feelings
is an act of self-compassion that creates trust. A daily ritual of
creative endeavors creates the time and space for expression of

emotions. Even if that time is initially not productive, by consistently making space for expression in an allowing, judgment-free, and unconditional way, creativity will begin to flow.

Sound and Music

Like the therapeutic use of writing and art, the use of sound and music is a powerful tool for accessing and releasing emotions that has been integral to every culture and spiritual tradition around the globe. Music and sound can be invaluable in balancing energy systems and maintaining harmony in our daily lives. The vibrational frequencies of harmonious sound waves interact positively with our own frequencies, influencing mental, emotional, spiritual, and physical states. When we talk about situations, words, or ideas "striking a chord" within us, we are referring to our innate musical nature, the experience of word-energies harmonizing with our own frequencies.

We have learned that our energy centers produce the same sound frequencies as the C scale. Indeed, researchers have found that when human cells are exposed to the sounds produced by various musical instruments, the most dramatic cellular response was observed from the sound of the human voice singing musical scales. Harmonious sounds from vocalizations, musical instruments, or recorded music help us transcend inner conflicts, move beyond ego self, and align with the frequency of our authentic selves—who we are at the core.

As we are inherently musical beings, music "tunes" our energy systems, harmonizing biological rhythms. Music can lower blood pressure, heart rate, and respiratory rate, synchronize brain waves, strengthen the immune response, release endorphins, relieve pain, and produce deep states of relaxation.

In *The Healing Power of Music: Recovery from Life-Threatening Illness Using Sound, Voice, and Music,* oncologist Mitchell Gaynor, M.D., tells the story of how he began using sound therapies in his allopathic practice after witnessing the transformational healing of patients who had received energy-based healing therapies. Dr. Gaynor writes, "I have long since come to accept nontraditional, holistic approaches as necessities, rather than potential options that must be integrated with the care and treatment of my patients."

I have also incorporated sound energy into my healing sessions. This has been particularly helpful when a client becomes overwhelmed from rapidly releasing emotional, physical, spiritual, or mental distress. In such situations, the introduction of a harmonious sound frequency into the healing environment has a dramatic and instantaneous effect. Striking a drum, singing bowl, or chime helps the client shift out of inner discordant frequencies and connects them to their essence by orienting to the harmonious vibration. The inclusion of sound therapy with hands-on energy healing techniques helps restore core energy flow through the nadis and chakra system, and can take the client into deeper levels of consciousness where they have access to inner resources.

Vocalizations are a powerful sound energy therapy technique, especially when combined with movement and deep breathing. Chanting, moaning, humming, and sighing, accompanied by deep breathing, can release the energetic effects of trauma and associated tension, pain, and emotion—particularly when intoning a sound on a single breath. Some clients spontaneously vocalize therapeutically during a healing session, but most feel inhibited and unconsciously avoid using their voice in this manner to prevent suppressed emotions from surfacing. Like other creative endeavors, being in a non-judging, unconditional state of mind allows vocal sounds to come through in a healing way.

Nora had been suffering from arrested grief after her brother's death. Although her phobia of driving on highways, her compulsive overeating, and her obsessive cleaning had all been alleviated with acutapping, she still had depressive episodes. In my energy assessment during one of these episodes, I found her frequencies to be very low. Her field was contracted with little energy flowing through her nadis and chakra system.

When I suggested Nora describe how she was feeling while I tapped on her acupoints, her voice was barely a whisper. After gaining her trust, I asked Nora if she could describe how she felt again, only this time putting more energy into her voice by speaking in a loud and melodramatic fashion, even if it felt silly. The moment that she did so, her energy began moving, followed by an emotional outburst, then a tingly sensation throughout her body, and finally a deep sense of peace.

After this experience, Nora began using vocalizations on her own to work with her grief. At first she reported that doing so felt awkward and the sounds she produced seemed stilted. But once she shifted her approach to one more playful in nature, and added deep breathing and movement, the vocalizations began to flow. As Nora surrendered to the experience, she was surprised at the sounds that came through her—deep moaning at first, and then grunting that became louder and more powerful, leaving her with a sense of lightness and clarity.

Although Nora no longer suffers from depression, she continues to play with sound energy therapies on a regular basis for self-care and balance.

Ritual and Ceremony

Another healing practice seen in spiritual traditions throughout history is the use of rituals and ceremony. Ritual and ceremony enhance spirituality and provide support through the healing process, particularly death, transition, and rebirth cycles. And it is through ritual and ceremony that we can integrate many everyday energy medicine measures into our lives, such as movement, sound, creativity, and deep breathing—healing the illusion of separation.

We are all familiar with ceremonies that honor beginnings, endings, and transitions, such as weddings, births, funerals, graduations, and religious coming-of-age rituals. The use of rituals and ceremonies is not confined to these events, however. Rituals and ceremonies can celebrate transitions in nature, such as seasonal solstices and the transitions from night to day and day to night. These rituals can also honor any beginning, ending, and transition in our lives, big or small. According to psychotherapist Steven Farmer, Ph.D., author of *Sacred Ceremony: How to Create Ceremonies for Healing, Transitions, and Celebrations*, "In the hectic and driven pace that has become a part of our modern, technologically dominated lives, it's even more critical that we access the spiritual realm consistently."

Morning rituals can include deep breathing while engaged in movement arts in sunlight, journaling, prayer, and setting intention. Our days can begin with consuming fresh water and raw food, and connecting with loved ones before starting our day. Similarly, evenings can include rituals that help us transition from the day's activities with gentle movement art practices, journaling, prayers, and re-connecting with loved ones before retiring for the night.

Ceremony has traditionally incorporated the four elements considered the foundation of life—earth, water, air, and fire. For example, the Native American "Sacred Smoke Bowl Blessing" ceremony, commonly known as "smudging," can include all four elements. Native Americans found that the smoke from burning herbs such as sage, cedar, sweetgrass, mugwort, or lavender had a detoxifying effect on energy, thus leaving people and places feeling clearer and lighter. To perform this ceremony, a lit candle can be used to ignite dried herbs placed in a seashell. A feather is commonly used to disburse the smoke from the burning herbs around a person or room. The herbs come from the Earth, the seashell from water. The feather represents air, and the candle fire.

Ceremony and ritual can also incorporate the use of a personal *altar*, creating sacred space in our homes and environments. Any space can be dedicated for use as an altar, and may contain objects that have spiritual, religious, and personal meaning. Altars can also feature representations of the four elements.

Creating ritual and ceremony was critical to my own healing. After years of failed infertility treatment cycles and early pregnancy losses, I felt like I was being crushed under a mountain of grief. My nose and eyes frequently watered with unexpressed tears, and my chest and shoulders ached with heaviness. It was through ceremony that I healed—a ceremony that became a ritual that carried me through successive losses. I established this ritual as my daily spiritual practice to process grief, create the space to grow a relationship with spirit, and heal the spiritual connection that felt missing in my life.

My ritual began with lighting a candle on an altar I had set up in a corner of our home. While listening to music I found cathartic, I opened my journal, took some slow, deep breaths, cleared my mind, and set intention for healing. This was my sacred time to grieve for the child I longed for, who I repeatedly lost as its life had barely begun.

When I first began this grieving ritual, I did not feel a spiritual connection for eleven days. But on the twelfth day, something changed. As I wrote in my journal, weeping along with the music and praying for my child's soul to be at peace, I heard a small voice in my mind.

"*What about your peace, dear mother?*"

Startled, I wrote in response in my journal, "How can I ever find peace when you are gone?"

"*I was never meant to stay. I came briefly to assist you along your journey and it was an honor to do so,*" came the response.

"I cannot go on without you."

"*You will grow. You will heal. You will find peace. These things I know. Let yourself cry until there are no more tears. And then rejoice at this healing, and dance with joy.*"

I did just that, weeping until the tears stopped. Then, getting up from the seat in front of my altar, I began moving to the music. With my eyes closed, I imagined myself joined by many women in white. We formed a circle, holding hands while we danced and chanted around a bonfire. I felt their presence and their support, and together we danced with the music until my sadness lifted. And in that moment, I found joy.

When trauma is released, when energy flow is restored, when frequencies harmonize and balance, the result is *joy*.

The Healing Journey

Although we have reached the end of this journey of healing through empowering information, the process goes on. Simply by reading this book, an opening has been created, movement is occurring, and a shift is taking place. You can continue this movement by exploring the resources in the recommended reading section, conducting your own personal research, playing with the concepts presented here, and drawing your own conclusions.

Your essential nature is to be whole. Within every ache and pain, every distressing emotion, every illness or disease—there is an opportunity to return to wholeness. There is an opportunity to take a deep breath, become aware of the message from your body-mind, observe with compassion ... and *heal.*

Even though I may feel overwhelmed by the many forms that everyday energy medicine can take, and think I have to do them all in order to do things "right," I am loveable and acceptable just as I am, and trust in my inner wisdom to know what is right for me. I know I can gradually incorporate changes into my life, one at a time, as I see fit.

Even though I may have been devalued by others at some point in my life, and used that experience as a model for devaluing myself, I love and accept myself, and now choose to fully value and nurture myself by integrating everyday energy medicine practices in my life.

APPENDIX

AN EXERCISE IN CONSCIOUS AND FOCUSED BREATHING

Make yourself comfortable, either lying down or sitting. If you are lying down, you may need a pillow under your knees to reduce pressure on your lower back, and a blanket in case you become chilled.

Let's begin with some slow, deep breaths, allowing your chest to rise, fall, and expand three-dimensionally—from top to bottom, side to side, and front to back. Slowly exhale until your lungs are completely empty. Don't push or force your lungs to do this—simply allow your expanded muscles and ribs to settle and drop completely. Then slowly inhale until your lungs are full. Notice any restriction as you do this.

As you continue, deepen and slow your rate of breathing, silently counting as you exhale and then inhale. How far can you count as you inhale? How far can you count as you exhale? Are they equal? As you relax, does the count get higher?

Now imagine that, as you exhale, you are breathing out anything negative—stress, angst, fear, and worries. These are all being released, all going out with your breath. And imagine that, as you inhale, you are taking in pure white light, the energy all around you.

You can continue with an inner mantra of: "Out with the

angst, in with the good." Or, "Out with the negative, in with the blessings." With each breath, you are sinking deeper and deeper into the chair or bed where you are sitting or lying. Your body may feel heavy.

As you continue deep breathing, scan your body head to toe. Take note of any place in your body that may feel tense, empty, or out of balance. Notice your head, your scalp, your face, your neck, your shoulders, your back, your chest, your arms, your belly, your pelvis, your legs. Where do you feel tense?

Imagine that you are sending your breath to this tense place in your body that feels empty or out-of-balance. And also imagine that you are surrounded by support to do this exercise. Continue observing what happens to that tension, without trying to make it go away, as you breathe slowly and deeply. You are a detached observer, with no purpose other than taking note of what happens.

Notice if the area of tension or emptiness you are focusing on has a shape or a color. Is it round, like a knot? What size? Is it flat like a band? If so, is it horizontal or vertical? You may notice that, as you focus on the area, it gets bigger or tighter. If it does, allow it to do so.

Continue sending your breath to this area as you observe without conditions. If this disrupted area were a pool of water, imagine slipping into it and lying in a state of surrender. If your mind wanders, gently bring yourself back to the area of disruption. Now what do you notice? Has the tension decreased? Is it gone? If not, continue the exercise until you notice a difference and feel relaxed.

In that state of relaxation, imagine that energy is flowing through your core, down through the center of your body in the same way that water flows through a garden hose. Imagine that flow of energy is steadily increasing and that you are connected to the source of that flow from the Earth, from the universe, and from God, as defined by you. You are one with everyone and everything. You are at peace. You are whole and complete, just as you are.

Acutapping

Refer to the following illustration of acupoints and the meridians they lie on to guide you in acutapping.

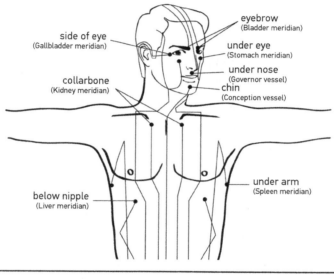

eyebrow
(Bladder meridian)

side of eye
(Gallbladder meridian)

under eye
(Stomach meridian)

under nose
(Governor vessel)

collarbone
(Kidney meridian)

chin
(Conception vessel)

under arm
(Spleen meridian)

below nipple
(Liver meridian)

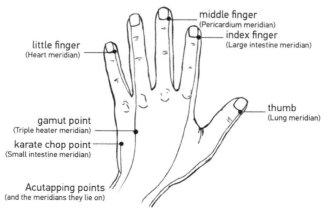

middle finger
(Pericardium meridian)

index finger
(Large intestine meridian)

little finger
(Heart meridian)

thumb
(Lung meridian)

gamut point
(Triple heater meridian)

karate chop point
(Small intestine meridian)

Acutapping points
(and the meridians they lie on)

The style and the specific acupoints used in the practice of acutapping (also known as EFT, or Emotional Freedom Technique) can vary—this is only a suggested technique offered for your personal use. If it varies from what you have seen elsewhere or what you have been taught, use whatever method works best for you or is your personal preference.

The meridians are labeled for your information. It is not necessary to know which are blocked to obtain results. Simply tap 5-7 times with the fingertip of the index finger of your dominant hand on all the points depicted in the illustration, while speaking or thinking about your issue.

The order of tapping does not matter, although it's easiest to progress down the body beginning with the eyebrow and ending at the hand. It does not matter which side of the body you tap on.

When you locate an acupoint on your body, it may feel sore to varying degrees.

Acutapping will not work if you are in a state of non-acceptance due to the energy reversal that self-rejection creates.

To correct a possible state of energy reversal, repeat three times that you accept yourself, or have the willingness and courage to entertain the possibility of accepting yourself, while tapping on the karate chop point. Or use the wording of the affirmations at the end of each chapter while tapping 5-7 times with your fingers on each point.

Pay attention to your body as you tap. You may notice a sense of relaxation, which may be accompanied by a feeling of lightness or a spontaneous deep breath. These are signs that an energy blockage has been released.

If you don't notice these signs and aren't sure how long you should tap, try tapping all the points 5-7 times each, repeating the cycle ten times total.

If you don't feel a change:

State that you accept yourself—even though you still have the issue or distress—while tapping on the karate chop point.

Try speaking loudly and melodramatically as you tap.

Take in a full breath at each tapping point, naming your distress as you exhale. (For example, if you are angry, while tapping on a point, take in a deep breath and say "I am angry" as you exhale.)

Recommended Reading

Art and Healing: Using Expressive Art to Heal Your Body, Mind, and Spirit by Barbara Ganim

Attachments: Why You Love, Feel and Act The Way You Do by Tim Clinton, Ed.D. and Gary Sibcy, Ph.D.

Becoming Attached: First Relationships and How They Shape Our Capacity to Love by Robert Karen, Ph.D.

Bee in Balance: A Guide to Healing the Whole Person with Honeybees, Oriental Medicine, and Common Sense by Amber Rose

Capturing the Aura: Integrating Science, Technology, and Metaphysics by C. E. Lindgren, D.Litt.

Chakra Foods for Optimal Health: A Guide to the Foods That Can Improve Your Energy, Inspire Creative Changes, Open Your Heart, and Heal Body, Mind, and Spirit by Deanna Minich, Ph.D.

Coming to Our Senses: Healing Ourselves and the World through Mindfulness by Jon Kabat-Zinn

Craniosacral Therapy and the Energetic Body: An Overview of Craniosacral Biodynamics by Roger Gilchrist

CranioSacral Therapy: Touchstone for Natural Healing by John E. Upledger, D.O., O.M.M.

Discovering The Body's Wisdom by Mirka Knaster

Dr. Mercola's Total Health Program: The Proven Plan to Prevent Disease and Premature Aging, Optimize Weight, and Live Longer by Joseph Mercola, M.D.

Energy Medicine: Balancing Your Body's Energies for Optimal Health, Joy, and Vitality by Donna Eden

Energy Medicine: Practical Applications and Scientific Proof by Norman Shealy, M.D., Ph.D.

Energy Medicine: The Scientific Basis by James Oschman, Ph.D.

Essential Reiki: A Complete Guide to an Ancient Healing Art by Diane Stein

Everyone's Guide to Homeopathic Medicines by Stephen Cummings, M.D., and Dana Ullman, M.P.H.

Everything You Need to Know to Feel Go(o)d by Candace B. Pert, Ph.D.

Flower Essences: Reordering Our Understanding and Approach to Illness and Health by Machaelle Small Wrigh

Free Your Breath, Free Your Life: How Conscious Breathing Can Relieve Stress, Increase Vitality, and Help You Live More Fully by Dennis Lewis

From Doctor to Healer: The Transformative Journey by Robbie David-Floyd, Ph.D. and Gloria St. John

Full Body Presence: Learning to Listen to Your Body's Wisdom by Suzanne Scurlock-Durana

Hands of Light: A Guide to Healing Through the Human Energy Field by Barbara Ann Brennan

Happiness: A Guide to Developing Life's Most Important Skill by Matthieu Ricard

Healing Back Pain: The Mind-Body Connection by John E. Sarno, M.D.

Healing Night: The Science and Spirit of Sleeping, Dreaming, and Awakening by Rubin Naiman, Ph.D.

Healing through Writing: A Journaling Guide to Emotional and Spiritual Growth by Anthony Parnell

Heal Your Body A-Z: The Mental Causes for Physical Illness and The Way to Overcome Them by Louise Hay

Last Child in the Woods: Saving Our Children from Nature Deficit Disorder by Richard Louv

Life Force: The Scientific Basis by Claude Swanson, Ph.D.

Light Emerging: The Journey of Personal Healing by Barbara Ann Brennan

Molecules of Emotion: The Science Behind Mind-Body Medicine by Candace B. Pert, Ph.D.

Outrageous Openness: Letting the Divine Take the Lead by Tosha Silver

Philosophy of Natural Therapeutics by Henry Lindlahr, M.D.

Play: How It Shapes the Brain, Opens the Imagination, and Invigorates the Soul by Stuart Brown, M.D.

Power Vs Force: The Hidden Determinants of Human Behavior by David R. Hawkins

Radical Forgiveness: A Revolutionary Five-State Process to Heal Relationships, Let Go of Anger and Blame, and Find Peace in Any Situation by Colin Tipping

Refrigerator Rights: Why We Need to Let People Into Our Hearts, Our Homes (and Our Refrigerators)...and How to Bring Even More Close Relationships Into Our Lives by Will Miller, Ed.D.

Sacred Ceremony: How to Create Ceremonies for Healing, Transitions, and Celebrations by Steven D. Farmer, Ph.D.

Spiritual Partnership: The Journey to Authentic Power by Gary Zukav

Tapping the Healer Within: Using Thought Field Therapy to Instantly Conquer Your Fears, Anxieties, and Emotional Distress by Roger J. Callahan, Ph.D.

The Attachment Parenting Book: A Commonsense Guide to Understanding and Nurturing Your Child by William Sears, M.D. and Martha Sears, R.N.

The Biology of Belief: Unleashing the Power of Consciousness, Matter & Miracles by Bruce H. Lipton, Ph.D.

The Body Remembers: The Psychophysiology of Trauma and Trauma Treatment by Babette Rothschild

The Complete Book of Water Healing by Dian Dincin Buchman, Ph.D.

The Dancing Wu Li Masters: An Overview of the New Physics by Gary Zukav

The Divided Mind: The Epidemic of Mindbody Disorders by John E. Sarno, M.D.

The Divine Matrix: Bridging Time, Space, Miracles, and Belief by Gregg Braden

The EFT Manual by Gary Craig

The Field: The Quest for the Secret Force of the Universe by Lynne McTaggart

The Gerson Therapy by Charlotte Gerson and Morton Walker

The Healing Power of Sound: Recovering from Life-Threatening Illness Using Sound, Voice, and Music by Mitchell Gaynor, M.D.

The Healing Sun: Sunlight and Health in the 21st Century by Richard Hobday, Ph.D.

The Heart of Christianity: Rediscovering a Life of Faith by Marcus J. Borg

The Heart's Code: Tapping the Wisdom and Power of Our Heart Energy by Paul Pearsall, Ph.D.

The Hidden Messages in Water by Masaru Emoto

The Intention Experiment: Using Your Thoughts to Change Your Life and the World by Lynne McTaggart

The Nature Principle: Human Restoration and the End of Nature-Deficit Disorder by Richard Louv

The Secret Life of Plants: A Fascinating Account of the Physical, Emotional, and Spiritual Relations Between Plants and Man by Peter Tompkins and Christopher Bird

The Sexual Healing Journey: A Guide for Survivors of Sexual Abuse by Wendy Maltz, M.S.W.

The Subtle Body: An Encyclopedia of Your Energetic Anatomy by Cyndi Dale

The Ultimate Healing System: The Illustrated Guide to Muscle Testing and Nutrition by Donald Lepore, N.D.

The Wellness Workbook: How to Achieve Enduring Health and Vitality by John Travis, M.D. and Regina Sara Ryan

Train Your Mind Change Your Brain: How a New Science Reveals Our Extraordinary Potential to Transform Ourselves by Sharon Begley

Transitions: Making Sense of Life's Changes by William Bridges

Trauma Energetics: A Study of Held-Energy Systems by William Redpath

Voices From the Womb by Michael Gabriel, M.A.

Waking the Tiger: Healing Trauma by Peter Levine, Ph.D.

Wheels of Light: Chakras, Auras, and the Healing Energy of the Body by Rosalyn Bruyere

FINAL THOUGHTS
& ACKNOWLEDGMENTS

"In my opinion, life's ultimate lesson is that we are
all here to help one another. My attitude, despite adversity,
will continue to remain fixed on the intention.
May yours remain fixed on your intention as well."

—DR. MATTHEW MCQUAID

AS I COME TO THE END of this book, I am almost overwhelmed with gratitude. I had nearly given up on the hope of writing another book after deciding not to publish my memoir. For over a year after that first failure, I found solace in helping plan my oldest son's wedding. But the day after the big event, I knew it was time to get back to my original intention.

After removing the wedding planning materials from my binder and replacing them with blank, lined paper, I recorded my intent to write a book at the top of the first page. But I had no idea what I was supposed to write about, other than the general topic of "healing."

In those first weeks, my attempts to get started were met with frustration and I felt overwhelmed. But when I let go and asked for help, things began to happen. I felt inspired to check online through Craigslist for assistance, and sure enough, I found an experienced professional writing consultant offering a writing-intensive workshop that very weekend.

Along the way, I had to throw out some of the "rules" I had taken in about writing, discard my outline, and pay more attention to my intuition. Regarding this intuitive process, author Gary Zukav writes, "Ideas began to occur to me that were not in my outlines. I left the outline behind and wrote about the new ideas. Eventually I realized I wasn't writing the book alone!" I too realized I was not writing this book alone.

As I focused my intention on writing to help others, the details of the book began to emerge from that desire. By being an open channel, the writing began to pour through me, taking shape and finding voice. Sources began appearing, one after another—books, clients, personal experiences, and insights.

As Jack Canfield, co-creator of the "Chicken Soup for the Soul" book series said in the film *The Secret*, "You can make it all the way from California to New York driving through the dark, because all you have to see is the next 200 feet—and that's how life tends to unfold before us, if we just trust…" Indeed, I only had to see the next step in my writing and trust that the following steps would unfold as I reached them.

What evolved was a book *about* the healing process, written *through* the healing process.

I can now see how every single experience in my life has led me to this moment, and I'm grateful for them all. The difficult events of my childhood, the years of infertility, and most recently the total knee replacement surgery that led me back to Western medicine to heal old wounds—all have brought me to this moment of perfect clarity.

Where do I begin thanking all those seen and unseen who have helped? My angels and spirit guides, you have been my constant companions throughout this process—carrying me through moments of doubt, fear, impatience, and frustration, and bringing me back to joy through your loving guidance.

To my beloved husband, Robert, through your love and your grounded, unwavering support, all things have been made possible. And to each of my children, Jonathan, Monica, and Jacob, and my daughter-in-law, Cyndi—thank you for your support and inspiration.

To my writing coach, David Hazard—from the moment I met you, I knew I could trust you. Thank you for believing in me, for "unpacking my head," and for holding the space for my healing process to unfold through the writing. You took me in directions I never would have thought of, and with gentleness, wisdom, and wit soothed my fears and helped with my organizational challenges.

Much gratitude goes to my first teacher, Kathleen Hanagan, for lighting the way when all seemed dark and I was lost. Your patient mentoring and guidance over nearly two decades made me the whole person I am today. And thank you also for your brilliant insight in suggesting the title of this book!

Thanks to my other teachers, Mary Branch Grove, Helen Yamada, and the late Chip Fortney, and the many professionals working in the healing arts who have played a role in my healing journey: the late Fred H. Mansbridge, Dale O'Brien, Christen McCormack, Donna Nichols, Sue Greer, Dr. Amber Rose, Carolyn Libby, Jan Iris Smith, Annie McFadden, Dr. John Wyrick, and Tully Hall.

To my first readers—my husband, Robert DuPree, my sister, Kristi Daly, my daughter, Monica DuPree, Rev. David Mosher, Anita Capizzi, R.N., and Marcia Keene, L.C.S.W.—your input was invaluable and greatly appreciated.

And I am grateful to all my wonderful clients whose stories were depicted in this book. You have all inspired me and it has been of the highest honor to work with each and every one of you.

I want to thank all those who came before me, the ancient healers whose wisdom has been passed down, and the many researchers of the last century who have bravely documented the science of healing and called for healthcare to return to nature in the face of fervent opposition.

And finally, I am grateful to you, dear reader, for taking the time to read this book, and for trusting me enough to explore what may be uncharted territory for you.

Namaste,

Heidi DuPree
September 2012

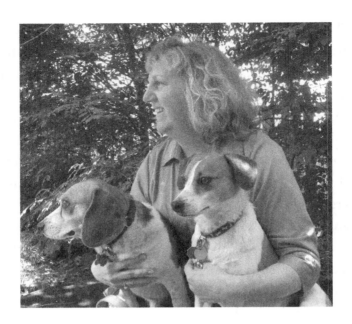

HEIDI DUPREE is an author, healing therapist,
holistic nurse, and Certified Traditional Naturopath with
over thirty years of experience in healthcare—half in
clinical nursing and half in energy medicine. For over
two decades she has avidly studied energy healing,
natural health, and the science of transformation. After
completing a Doctorate in Traditional Naturopathy,
she became certified by the American Naturopathic
Certification Board. Heidi is also an ordained nonde-
nominational healing minister, and a musician. She lives
in Ashburn, Virginia with her husband, Robert, youngest
son, Jacob, two dogs, and two cats.

To download a Reading Group Guide,
and receive a free Energy Medicine Kit
for Healing and Integration, visit
www.HeidiDuPree.com